A Concise Guide to HIPAA Compliance

An Easy-to-Follow Guide Derived From Official Government Sources

Apex Legal Publishing
Akron, Ohio

Second Edition

Copyright © 2020 Apex Legal Publishing

All rights reserved

ISBN: 9781708924799

First Edition © 2019 Apex Legal Publishing

Contents

1. Introduction

This HIPAA Compliance Guide has been compiled for the benefit of administrators and managers who are aware that they have to become HIPAA compliant, but are unsure of what is involved and need to develop a better understanding of HIPAA rules and regulations. The guide should also be of use to businesses that are considering providing services to healthcare organizations that will require contact with electronic protected health information (PHI) and compliance with HIPAA.

Understanding HIPAA is not easy. Current legislation is comprised of the original 1996 Healthcare Insurance Portability and Accountability Act with additional sections added via the Privacy Rule of 2000, the Security Rule of 2003, the Health Information Technology for Economic and Clinical Health Act (HITECH) and the American Recovery and Reinvestment Act introduced in 2009 (ARRA).

The Omnibus Final Rule of 2013 enacted further legislation within HIPAA and more changes to the guidelines for protecting patient healthcare and payment information are anticipated in the future as the Meaningful Use incentive program progresses and further HIPAA audits are conducted by the US Department of Health and Human Services´ Office for Civil Rights (OCR).

HIPAA legislation is so far-reaching, and covers so many different scenarios, that our intention for this HIPAA Compliance Guide is to provide an extensive outline of what hospital administrators and practice managers need to know before implementing measures to comply with HIPAA.

To recreate multiple HIPAA-related scenarios — and illustrate how HIPAA applies in each — would be confusing and counter-productive. Consequently, we have broken down this HIPAA Compliance Guide into seven separate sections for ease of navigation. This guide should serve as the foundation for more focused research, depending on the business nature of the organization or practice.

2. The Background and Objectives of HIPAA

The Healthcare Insurance Portability and Accountability Act (HIPAA) was signed into law on 21st August 1996 as an Act to "improve the portability and accountability of health insurance coverage" for employees between jobs, and to combat waste, fraud and abuse in health insurance and healthcare delivery. The Act also contained passages to promote the use of medical savings accounts by introducing tax breaks, provide coverage for employees with pre-existing medical conditions and the simplification of the administration of health insurance.

The procedures for simplifying the administration of health insurance became a vehicle for encouraging the healthcare industry to computerize patients´ medical records. This particular part of the Act spawned the Health Information Technology for Economic and Clinical Health Act (HITECH) in 2009, which in turn lead to the introduction of the Meaningful Use incentive program. The HITECH Act was described by leaders in the healthcare industry as "the most important piece of healthcare legislation to be passed in the last 20 to 30 years".

Development of the HIPAA Privacy and Security Rules

Once HIPAA had been signed into law, the US Department of Health and Human Services set about creating the first HIPAA Privacy and Security Rules. The Privacy Rule had an effective compliance date of April 14, 2003 and defined Protected Health Information (PHI) as "any information held by a covered entity which concerns health status, the provision of healthcare, or payment for healthcare that can be linked to an individual". The full list of personal identifiers that are considered to be "linked to an individual" and make health information PHI can be found in the section of this page dedicated to the HIPAA Privacy Rule.

The Privacy Rule set standards covering the allowable uses and disclosures of PHI and under what circumstances it is possible. These are often referred to as HIPAA TPO uses and disclosures as they are related to the provision of Treatment, payment for healthcare, and for healthcare operations. The Privacy Rule placed restrictions on the use of PHI for marketing, fundraising, and research. These uses are not prohibited, but these uses and disclosures are only permissible if prior authorization has been obtained in writing from the patient or their designated representative. Patients were also given the right to withhold information about treatment from health insurance providers if that treatment was privately funded.

The HIPAA Security Rule came into force two years later on April 21, 2005. The Security Rule deals specifically with electronically stored PHI (ePHI) and stipulated three classes of safeguards were required for ePHI – administrative, physical and technical – to ensure the confidentiality, integrity, and availability of ePHI. These safeguards had the following goals:

- ❖ Administrative– To create policies and procedures designed to clearly show how the entity will comply with the act.

- ❖ Physical– To control physical access to areas of data storage to protect against inappropriate access.

- ❖ Technical– To protect communications containing PHI when transmitted electronically over open networks and for data at rest.

The HIPAA Enforcement Rule

The failure of many covered entities to fully comply with the HIPAA Privacy and Security Rules resulted in the introduction of the Enforcement Rule in March 2006. The Enforcement Rule gave the Department of Health and Human Services the power to investigate complaints against covered entities that were failing to comply with the Privacy Rule and to fine covered entities for avoidable breaches of ePHI due to not implementing appropriate safeguards to comply with the HIPAA Security Rule.

The HHS' Office for Civil Rights was also given the power to bring criminal charges against persistent offenders who fail to introduce corrective measures within 30 days of a breach or discovery of a HIPAA violation.

The HITECH Act of 2009 and the HIPAA Breach Notification Rule

The introduction of the Health Information Technology for Economic and Clinical Health (HITECH) Act in 2009 had the primary goal of compelling healthcare authorities to use Electronic Health Records (EHRs). The HITECH Act called for the creation of the Meaningful Use incentive program. Stage one of Meaningful Use was rolled out the following year which incentivized healthcare organizations to maintain PHI in electronic format rather than in paper files and other physical formats through financial payment for achieving the core objectives and a selection of other meaningful uses of EHRs.

With the incentive program also came an extension of HIPAA Rules to include business associates and third-party suppliers to the healthcare industry. The HITECH Act also triggered the creation of the HIPAA Breach Notification Rule which stipulated that all affected individuals must be notified of a breach of their PHI within 60 days of discovery of the breach.

The HIPAA Breach Notification Rule also required all breaches of unsecured ePHI affecting more than 500 individuals to be reported to the Department of Health and Human Services' Office for Civil Rights within 60 days of the discovery of a breach. Breaches involving fewer than 500 healthcare records must also be reported, although covered entities are only required to do this annually within 60 days of the end of the year in which the breach was experienced. The criteria for reporting breaches of ePHI were subsequently extended in the Omnibus Final Rule of March 2013.

The Omnibus Final Rule of 2013

The most recent legislation to change HIPAA was the Omnibus Final Rule of 2013. The rule barely introduced any new legislation, instead it closed gaps in existing HIPAA and HITECH regulations – for example, specifying the encryption standards that need to be applied to render ePHI unusable, undecipherable and unreadable in the event of a breach.

Many definitions were amended or added to clear up grey areas – for example the definition of "Workforce" was changed to make it clear that the term includes employees, volunteers, trainees, and other persons whose conduct, in the performance of work for a covered entity or business associate, is under the direct control of the covered entity or business associate.

The HIPAA Privacy and Security Rules were also amended to allow patient health information to be held indefinitely (the previous legislation had stipulated it should be held for fifty years) and to apply new penalties – as dictated by the HITECH Act – to covered entities that were found not to have complied with the requirements of HIPAA.

Amendments were also included to account for changing work practices brought about by technological advances, with the Final Rule covering the use of mobile devices in particular. A significant number of healthcare professionals are now using their own mobile devices to access and communicate ePHI, and the Omnibus Final Rule included new administrative procedures and policies to account for this and update HIPAA to cover scenarios which could not have been foreseen in 1996.

Effects of the Omnibus Final Rule

What the Omnibus Final Rule achieved more than any other previous legislation was to make covered entities more aware of HIPAA safeguards that they had to implement. Many healthcare organizations – who had been in breach of HIPAA for almost two decades – implemented new measures to comply with the regulations, such as using data encryption on portable devices and computer networks, implementing secure messaging solutions for internal communications with care teams and installing more robust firewalls and multi-layered network security defenses.

The financial penalties resulting from data breaches along with the colossal costs of issuing breach notifications, providing credit monitoring services, and conducting damage mitigation makes investment in new technology to protect healthcare data not only efficient, but also cost-effective.

The HIPAA Compliance Audit Program

In 2011, the Office for Civil Rights commenced a series of pilot compliance audits to assess how well healthcare providers were implementing the HIPAA Privacy, Security and Breach Notification Rules. The first round of audits was completed in 2012 and highlighted the dire state of HIPAA compliance.

Audited organizations registered numerous violations of the HIPAA Breach Notification Rule, HIPAA Privacy Rule, and HIPAA Security Rule, with the latter resulting in the highest number of violations. OCR issued action plans and technical guidance to help those organizations achieve compliance.

The second round of compliance audits in 2017 focused on the most problematic areas of compliance for healthcare providers. The ultimate goal of OCR is to run a permanent compliance audit program, and it has taken great strides towards this goal in the following months. OCR implemented a new web portal which streamlined the collection of audit documentation, freeing up resources that will allow it to conduct more audits in the future.

The age of lax security standards has now passed and the healthcare industry, like the financial industry before it, must now raise data security standards to ensure healthcare data remains private and confidential.

Any covered entity which does not implement the required controls now faces severe financial penalties, sanctions, and a potential loss of license to practice. Criminal proceedings can also be initiated for failing to secure PHI and for other willful violations of HIPAA Rules.

HIPAA Pilot Audit Findings

- ❖ 2/3 of audited entities had not completed a full and accurate risk analysis

- ❖ 980 compliance issues were identified

- ❖ Only 13 entities had no negative findings

- ❖ Healthcare providers accounted for 65% of negative findings but constituted 53% of the audit set

- ❖ 1/3 of all violations resulted from ignorance of HIPAA requirements

- ❖ 58 out of 59 providers had at least one finding

- ❖ Data security was the basis for 60% of findings but constituted only 28% of the possible total

- ❖ Privacy Rule violations accounted for 30% of negative findings; 10% were due to breach notification violations

- ❖ Small organizations demonstrated problems with all aspects of HIPAA compliance

---

3. The Administrative Simplification Rules

One of the main aims of HIPAA was to simplify the administration of healthcare and improve efficiency. Prior to the introduction of HIPAA, healthcare organizations, including providers and health plans, often used different code sets.

While these code sets worked fine internally, without standard code sets and rules, conducting healthcare transactions such as verifying eligibility, enrolling and disenrolling new patients/plan members, coordinating benefits, and billing was unnecessarily complex and inefficient.

Medical billing and electronic payments were introduced in the 1980's and 1990s. Electronic transactions are faster and more efficient and allow payments to be processed much more quickly; however, the healthcare industry was not getting the full benefits of automation due to a lack of operating standardization across the healthcare industry.

It was clear that there was a need to standardize transactions and for national identifiers and standard code sets to be introduced. These are all covered by the HIPAA Administrative Simplification Rules.

The HIPAA Administrative Simplification Rules must be followed by all healthcare providers, health plans, and healthcare clearinghouses that conduct healthcare transactions electronically. Standards are set for electronic transactions to ensure uniformity when communicating information.

There is no requirement for healthcare organizations to transition to electronic health records and transactions – although incentives are offered through the Meaningful Use program – but when healthcare transactions are conducted electronically, it is necessary to comply with the HIPAA Administrative Simplification Rules.

The HIPAA Administrative Simplification Rules include:

❖ Electronic transaction standards;

❖ Standard code sets; and

❖ Unique identifiers

Standards and code sets are detailed in the Health Insurance Portability and Accountability Act (HIPAA) of 1996 but were updated by the Patient Protection and Affordable Care Act (ACA). The latter introduced new operating rules to standardize business practices to further improve efficiency in healthcare.

While transitioning to new code sets and adopting new standards can cause headaches, ultimately the change will reduce time spent on paperwork and lessen the administrative burden on providers. Adoption of the standards leads to substantial cost savings and allows providers to spend more time giving are to patients.

Electronic Transaction Standards

Transactions are any electronic exchange of information between two parties for the purpose of carrying out activities related to the provision of healthcare, including financial and administrative activities.

The transactions covered by the HIPAA Administrative Simplification Rules include the following types of transactions:

- ❖ Claims and encounter information
- ❖ Payment and remittance advice
- ❖ Claims status
- ❖ Eligibility
- ❖ Enrollment and disenrollment
- ❖ Referrals and authorizations
- ❖ Coordination of benefits
- ❖ Premium payment

All the above transactions require covered entities to use an adopted standard from ASC X12N or, for certain pharmacy transactions, NCPDP.

Since ACA was signed into law, standards must be adopted for the electronic transfer of funds and electronic healthcare claims attachments. New operating rules were also set for each of the existing covered transactions, and a standard identifier had to be adopted by health plans. ACA also introduced new financial penalties for organizations found not to be in compliance with the HIPAA Administrative Simplification standards and operating rules.

Code Sets

HIPAA requires all covered entities to adopt specific code sets for diagnoses and procedures, which must be used in all transactions. Code sets are necessary as they inform a wide range of healthcare functions.

The code sets ensure all covered entities use standard codes for diagnoses, procedures, treatments, diagnostic tests, and equipment and supplies.

The code sets detailed in HIPAA include:

- ❖ The 10th Edition of the International classification of Diseases (ICD-10)
- ❖ Current Procedure Terminology (CPT)
- ❖ Healthcare Common Procedure Coding System (HCPCS)
- ❖ Code on Dental Procedures and Nomenclature (CDT)
- ❖ National Drug Codes (NDC)

Unique identifiers

All HIPAA covered entities are required to use unique identifiers for plan members, employees, and providers. There is no current national identifier for patients. The identifiers are:

- ❖ Health Plan Identifier (HPID)
- ❖ National Provider Identifier (NPI)
- ❖ An Employer Identifier Number (EIN)

It is a requirement of HIPAA for NPIs and EINs to be used on all HIPAA transactions.

Compliance and Enforcement of the Administrative Simplification Rules

While the Department of Health and Human Services' Office for Civil Rights is responsible for issuing guidance and enforcing compliance with the HIPAA Privacy, Security, and Breach Notification Rules, the administration and enforcement of compliance with the HIPAA Administrative Simplification Rules is the responsibility of the HHS' Centers for Medicare & Medicaid Services, irrespective of whether providers accept Medicare or Medicaid.

In 2019, the CMS commenced a series of audits to assess compliance with the HIPAA Administrative Simplification Rules. Random audits will be conducted on a range of different HIPAA-covered entities to ensure they are adhering to the HIPAA Administrative Simplification Rules standards.

4. The Privacy Rule

❖ The HIPAA Privacy Rule

❖ "PHI" Defined

❖ Uses and Disclosures of PHI

❖ HIPAA Authorizations

❖ De-identification of Protected Health Information

❖ Marketing and Fundraising Protocols

❖ Patient Access to Medical Records

❖ Designated Record Sets

❖ Charging for Copies of PHI

❖ Amendments to Healthcare Records

❖ Accounting of Disclosures of PHI

❖ Notices of Privacy Practices

The HIPAA Privacy Rule

"The HIPAA Privacy Rule establishes national standards to protect individuals' medical records and other personal health information and applies to health plans, healthcare clearinghouses, and those healthcare providers that conduct certain healthcare transactions electronically. The Rule requires appropriate safeguards to protect the privacy of personal health information, and sets limits and conditions on the uses and disclosures that may be made of such information without patient authorization. The Rule also gives patients' rights over their health information, including rights to examine and obtain a copy of their health records and to request corrections"

Definition provided by the US Department of Health and Human Services

The HIPAA Privacy Rule regulates the use and disclosure of Protected Health Information (PHI) held by covered entities and business associates – Third-party service providers who are provided with PHI in order to perform services and vendors whose products and services come into contact with PHI.

What constitutes "PHI" is broadly regarded to be any part of an individual's medical records or payment history and. To provide a more comprehensive definition of "PHI" for those who have a responsibility to protect it, we have dedicated an entire section to "What is PHI?" below.

For the purposes of this section, a covered entity is an individual or organization that conducts healthcare transactions electronically. This is likely to include healthcare providers, health plans and healthcare clearinghouses; although some exceptions exist to this generalization.

The Privacy Rule requires covered entities to notify individuals about how their PHI will be used. Covered entities must also keep track of disclosures of PHI and document their privacy policies and procedures. They must appoint a privacy officer and a contact person responsible for receiving complaints and training all members of the workforce about the policies and procedures regarding PHI. In particular, the HIPAA privacy officer must provide training on when PHI can be disclosed, to whom, and under what specific circumstances.

A covered entity may disclose PHI to facilitate treatment, payment or healthcare operations without a patient's express written authorization. Any other disclosures of PHI require the covered entity to obtain written authorization from the individual before their PHI is used. When a covered entity discloses any PHI, it must make a reasonable effort to disclose only the minimum necessary information to achieve the required purpose.

Covered entities may disclose protected health information to law enforcement officials for law enforcement purposes (including court orders, court-ordered warrants and subpoenas), although care must still be taken before that information is disclosed. Recently, a medical facility was found to have been negligent for disclosing PHI without first informing the patient (a court ruled that federal law superseded a county-issued subpoena).

In addition to protecting the privacy of individuals, the Privacy Rule aims to make it easier for patients to access their medical information. The Privacy Rule requires covered entities to provide a copy of a patient's healthcare data within 30 days of receiving a written request. They must also disclose PHI, as required by law, in cases of suspected child abuse in order to allow the state child welfare agencies to identify or locate a suspect, fugitive, material witness or missing person.

The Privacy Rule gives individuals the right to request that a covered entity corrects any inaccurate PHI. It also requires covered entities to take reasonable steps to ensure the confidentiality of communications with individuals. An individual who believes that the Privacy Rule is not being upheld can file a complaint with the Department of Health and Human Services' Office for Civil Rights.

NOTE: The HIPAA Privacy Rule applies to PHI in any form. This includes computer and paper files, x-rays, physician appointment schedules, medical bills, dictated notes, conversations, and information entered into patient portals.

"PHI" Defined

As mentioned above, PHI stands for protected health information and is defined as "any information held by a covered entity which concerns health status, the provision of healthcare, or payment for healthcare that can be linked to an individual". But what is this "information" and who does it apply to?

HIPAA regulations list eighteen different personal identifiers which, when linked with health information are classed as protected health information. If any one of the identifiers below is linked to health information, it is considered to be PHI.

The eighteen personal identifiers are:

- ❖ Names
- ❖ All geographical data smaller than a state
- ❖ Dates (other than year) directly related to an individual
- ❖ Telephone numbers
- ❖ Fax numbers
- ❖ Email addresses
- ❖ Social Security numbers
- ❖ Medical record numbers
- ❖ Health insurance plan beneficiary numbers
- ❖ Account numbers
- ❖ Certificate/license numbers
- ❖ Vehicle identifiers and serial numbers including license plates
- ❖ Device identifiers and serial numbers
- ❖ Web URLs
- ❖ Internet protocol (IP) addresses
- ❖ Biometric identifiers (i.e. retinal scan, fingerprints, Etc.)
- ❖ Full face photos and comparable images
- ❖ Any unique identifying number, characteristic or code

Entities Required to Protect PHI

Persons with a responsibility to protect PHI and comply with the HIPAA Privacy Rule fall into three main categories – Covered entities, business associates, and subcontractors used by business associates.

Covered entities are the individuals, institutions or organizations that maintain patient healthcare or payment information or would reasonably be expected to come into contact with PHI in the course of their daily duties, mainly healthcare providers, health plans and healthcare clearinghouses. Examples of covered entities include:

Healthcare Providers – Healthcare providers include all "providers of services" (e.g., institutional providers such as hospitals) and "providers of medical or health services" (e.g., non-institutional providers such as physicians, dentists and other practitioners) as defined by Medicare, and any other person or organization that furnishes, bills, or receives payment for the provision of healthcare services.

Health Plans – Individual and group health plans that provide or pay the cost of medical care are covered entities.Health plans include health, dental, vision, and prescription drug insurers, health maintenance organizations ("HMOs"), Medicare, Medicaid, Medicare+ Choice and Medicare supplement insurers and long-term care insurers (excluding nursing home fixed-indemnity policies). Health plans also include some employer-sponsored group health plans, government and church-sponsored health plans and multi-employer health plans.

Healthcare Clearinghouses – Healthcare clearinghouses include billing services, repricing companies, community health management information systems and value-added networks that perform clearinghouse functions; such as processing non-standard information they receive from another entity into a standard version, or vice versa.

In most instances, healthcare clearinghouses will receive individually identifiable health information only when they are providing these processing services to a health plan or healthcare provider as a business associate. In such instances, only certain provisions of the Privacy Rule are applicable to healthcare clearinghouses' uses and disclosures of protected health information.

Business Associates – business associates are persons or entities that are not employed by a covered entity but perform or assist in performing tasks on behalf of a covered entity that involve contact with PHI. A member of a covered entity's workforce is not one of its business associates, but a covered entity could in theory be a business associate of another covered entity, depending on the services it provides.

Business associate functions or activities on behalf of a covered entity include claims processing, data analysis, utilization reviews, billing services, data storage services, cloud and hosting services. Software providers are also considered business associates if the software comes into contact with ePHI.

Business associate services to a covered entity are limited to legal, actuarial, accounting, consulting, data aggregation, management, administrative, accreditation or financial services.

Persons or organizations are not considered business associates if their functions or services do not involve the use or disclosure of protected health information, and where any access to PHI by such persons would be incidental, if at all.

Business associates — and independent contractors or subcontractors who are likely to have access to PHI to perform tasks for the business associate — include labs and lab technicians, collection agencies, message and confirmation services, IT and technical personnel, and non-employed consultants.

Covered entities engaging in business transactions with business associates — who will encounter PHI in the course of the business transaction — must ensure that a "business associate agreement" is in place before any PHI is provided or accessed by the business associate. Details of business associate agreements and how they are applied appear in the "How HIPAA is Enforced?" section of this document.

Uses and Disclosures of PHI

The HIPAA Privacy Rule limits how PHI can be used and disclosed to protect healthcare and payment information while attempting to avoid the creation of unnecessary barriers that could impact the delivery of healthcare services.

The HIPAA Privacy Rule generally prohibits a covered entity from using or disclosing PHI unless authorized by patients, except where this prohibition would interfere with delivery of quality healthcare or with certain other important public benefits or national priorities.

Both access to treatment and efficient payment for healthcare services requires the use and disclosure of PHI and is essential to the effective operation of the healthcare system. In addition, certain healthcare operations—such as administrative, financial, legal, and quality improvement activities—conducted by or on behalf of healthcare providers and health plans – are essential for the provision of medical services to patients and for processing payments.

Many individuals expect PHI to be used and disclosed, as necessary, for providing treatment, and to some extent, to ensure a covered entity's healthcare business can operate efficiently. To avoid interfering with an individual's access to quality healthcare or the efficient payment for healthcare services, the HIPAA Privacy Rule permits a covered entity to use and disclose protected health information, with certain limits and protections, for treatment, payment and healthcare operations activities – Often referred to as HIPAA TPO activities.

Application of the Use and Disclosure Criteria

The full criteria for what constitutes a "use" or a "disclosure" of PHI are exceptionally long (see HIPAA Privacy Rule §45 CFR 164.501 onward). In certain circumstances, the disclosure of PHI is allowed without consent; but for the sake of brevity, we have listed the occasions when a covered entity can use or disclose PHI without first obtaining the patient´s consent.

A covered entity may, without the individual's authorization, use or disclose PHI for treatment, payment or the provision of healthcare operations under the following scenarios:

- ❖ A hospital may use PHI about an individual to provide healthcare to the individual and may consult with other healthcare providers about the individual's treatment

- ❖ A healthcare provider may disclose PHI about an individual as part of a claim for payment to a health plan

- ❖ A health plan may use PHI to provide customer service to its enrollees

- ❖ A covered entity may disclose PHI for the treatment activities of any healthcare provider (including providers not covered by the HIPAA Privacy Rule). For example:

- ❖ A primary care provider may send a copy of an individual's medical records to a specialist who needs the information to provide treatment

- ❖ A hospital may send a patient's healthcare instructions during a patient transfer to a nursing home

- ❖ A covered entity may disclose PHI to another covered entity or a healthcare provider (including providers not covered by the Privacy Rule) for the payment activities of the entity that receives the information. For example:

- ❖ A physician may send an individual's health plan coverage information to a laboratory to bill for patient services it provided

- ❖ A hospital emergency department may give a patient's payment information to an ambulance service provider to request payment for transportation services

HIPAA Authorizations

Prior to any use or disclosure of an individual's protected health information that is not permitted by the HIPAA Privacy Rule, written authorization must be obtained from the individual. A HIPAA authorization is a detailed written document that authorizes a covered entity to use or disclose an individual's protected health information for the specific purposes outlined in the authorization form.

An authorization is generally required for any use or disclosure that falls outside the definition of treatment, payment, or healthcare operations.

There are several required elements for authorization forms. They must include:

- ❖ Meaningful and specific information about the uses and disclosures that the patient is authorizing

- ❖ The name or details of the class of person authorized to use or disclose PHI and the name or class of person to whom the information will be disclosed.

❖ The purpose of the use or disclosure

❖ The time frame that the authorization covers, including an expiry date.

❖ The individual's signature and the date that the authorization was given

The individual must also be notified on the form that they have the right to revoke the authorization by submitting a request in writing together with either:

❖ Exceptions to the right to revoke and details of how the right to revoke the authorization can be exercised; or

❖ The extent to which that information is detailed in the organization's notice of privacy practices.

The authorization must also state the ability or inability to condition treatment, payment, enrollment, or eligibility for benefits on the authorization.

The HIPAA "Minimum Necessary" Standard

The HIPAA Privacy Rule stipulates the allowable uses and disclosures of identifiable protected health information but there is also a restriction placed on how much PHI can be accessed or disclosed as detailed in the HIPAA minimum necessary standard.

The HIPAA minimum necessary standard limits uses, disclosures, and requests for PHI to the minimum amount necessary to achieve the desired purpose. The minimum necessary standard applies to PHI in all forms, including physical records, electronic PHI, and verbal disclosures of PHI.

The HIPAA minimum necessary standard applies to all uses and disclosures of PHI and ePHI, which includes disclosures to other HIPAA covered entities, PHI access by healthcare employees, and disclosures of PHI to business associates.

A covered entity is required to develop policies and procedures that reasonably limit its uses, disclosures, and requests for protected health information. It is up to the covered entity to determine how much PHI is required to achieve a particular purpose.

Under this standard, a covered entity is required to develop role-based access policies and procedures that limit which members of its workforce may have access to protected health information for treatment, payment and healthcare operations and the amount of PHI that can be accessed.

There are a limited number of exceptions where the HIPAA minimum standard does not apply.

These are:

❖ Disclosures to a healthcare provider for the purpose of treating patients and requests from healthcare providers for PHI for treatment purposes.

- ❖ Disclosures to an individual who is exercising the right to access or obtain a copy of their healthcare information that is part of a designated record set, apart from psychotherapy notes, and PHI that has been compiled for civil, criminal, or administrative actions or proceedings.

- ❖ A use of disclosure pursuant to a valid authorization

- ❖ Uses and disclosures that are required by law

- ❖ Disclosures to the HHS as detailed in 45 CFR Part 160 Subpart C

- ❖ Uses and disclosures that are required in order to comply with HIPAA regulations

De-identification of Protected Health Information

The HIPAA Privacy Rule places restrictions on uses and disclosures of identifiable protected health information, but if health information is stripped of all information that allows an individual to be identified, secondary uses of that information are permitted, such as the provision of the information to organizations for research purposes.

The HIPAA Privacy Rule stipulates two methods that can be used to de-identify protected health information: Expert Determination and the Safe Harbor method.

Expert determination requires a person with appropriate experience and knowledge of generally accepted statistical and scientific principles and techniques for removing individually identifiable information to apply those principles and methods and determine that the risk of an individual being identified from the data is very small, either using the information alone or in combination with other information that is reasonably available. The methods used and the results of any analyses must be documented and must justify the determination.

The safe harbor method involves the removal of all 18 types of identifiers detailed in the "What is PHI" section of this guide.

When either of these approaches is used, PHI is no longer identifiable and is no longer protected by the HIPAA Privacy Rule.

Marketing and Fundraising Limitations

Restrictions on the use of PHI for Marketing

As you might expect, HIPAA regulations strictly limit what can be done with PHI beyond the standard permitted uses and disclosures. For example, the Privacy Rule expressly prohibits covered entities from selling PHI to third parties and using PHI for marketing activities without prior patient authorization.

The regulations state that if a covered entity receives "financial remuneration" for communicating treatment or operational information to advertise a third-party product or service, then prior authorization must be obtained from the individual. With some limited exceptions, business associates are prohibited from using PHI for their own purposes.

Refill reminders or other communications about a currently prescribed drug for an individual, including self-administered drugs or biologics (such as insulin pumps) are excluded from this prohibition, but only if any received financial remuneration is reasonably related to the cost of making the communication.

Face to face marketing, including the handing out of written materials such as pamphlets and promotional gifts of nominal value, are also excluded from the authorization requirement so as not to intrude into the doctor-patient relationship and also so that healthcare providers can leave general circulation materials in their offices for patients to pick up during their visits.

Additionally, a communication that is made for the following treatment and healthcare operations purposes, where no financial remuneration is received, are also excluded from this prohibition:

❖ For the treatment of an individual by a healthcare provider or to direct or recommend alternative treatments, therapies, healthcare providers or settings of care to the individual

❖ To describe a health-related product or service (or payment for such product or service) that is provided by or is included in a plan – including communications about healthcare provider or health plan networks, enhancements to a health plan, and health-related products or services available only to health plan participants that add value to, but are not part of, an existing plan

❖ For case management or care coordination, contacting of individuals with information about treatment alternatives and related functions if these activities do not fall within the definition of treatment.

Financial remuneration is defined as "direct or indirect payment from or on behalf of a third party whose product or service is being described" other than payment for treatment of an individual. "Financial remuneration" does not include non-financial benefits, such as in-kind benefits provided in exchange for making a communication about a product or service. If a covered entity is currently sending marketing materials to its participants – or is allowing service providers or vendors to do so through its website – the marketing practices should be evaluated to ensure they are in compliance with the HIPAA Privacy Rule.

Restrictions on Disclosure and Sale of PHI for "Fundraising" Purposes

The Omnibus Final Rule of 2013 further clarified the HITECH Act's prohibition of the sale of PHI. Under the Omnibus Rule, the sale of PHI generally means a disclosure of PHI if a covered entity receives direct or indirect remuneration from or on behalf of the recipient in exchange for the PHI. It is not necessary for a covered entity to transfer ownership of the PHI for the transaction to constitute a "sale."

The Omnibus Final Rule expands the definition of PHI that may be used for fundraising purposes (with patient authorization) to include demographic information relating to the individual – including name, address, other contact information, age, gender and date of birth; dates that healthcare was provided to the individual; information about the general department of treatment (e.g., cardiology, oncology, pediatrics, etc.); the treating physician; outcome information and health insurance status.

If a covered entity uses PHI for authorized fundraising purposes, it must still ensure that only the necessary amount of PHI is used or disclosed. A clear and explicit opt-out must be included with all fundraising communications; however, covered entities are free to decide what methods individuals can use to opt out of future fundraising communications – provided the method does not constitute an undue burden on an individual.

Please note that any use of PHI for marketing or fundraising must be consistent with a covered entity's "Notice of Privacy Practices" – a subject that is addressed later in our HIPAA Compliance Guide.

Patient Access to Medical Records

The HIPAA Privacy Rule has always provided individuals with the right to access and obtain copies of health information maintained in provider or health plan records. Under the existing regulations, when a patient makes such a request, the covered entity has up to 30 days to provide the requested access or a copy of the requested data; however, the provider or plan can take up to an additional 60 days if the information requested is stored off-site.

Patients can be charged a reasonable, cost-based fee for copies of their information, to cover the cost of both labor and supplies. This right of access has been part of the Privacy Rule since it was first implemented; although many patients have faced obstacles when trying to obtain copies of their health information.

The Privacy Rule covers identifiable health information in both paper and digital form, so this right of patient access has always applied to all forms of PHI. However, in the HITECH Act, Congress made it clear that when a patient's information is stored electronically, patients have the right to obtain an electronic copy and to have that copy sent, at their request, to another person or entity, such as a doctor, caregiver, their personal representative, or a personal health record or mobile health app.

New regulations enacted by the Omnibus Final Rule implement this mandate and also clarify how this right to digital data can be exercised. Patients have the right to an electronic copy "in the form or format they request" – but only if the provider or plan is capable of producing the copy in the requested format. If the data isn't "readily producible" in the format requested by the patient, the provider – or plan – and the patient are expected to come to an agreement on an alternative acceptable, machine-readable digital format.

The new rules still allow healthcare providers and health plans to ask patients to submit written requests for copies of their health information, although this is not a requirement of the Privacy Rule. However, if the patient wants to have the electronic copy transmitted directly to a third party, the new rules require that this type of request must be in writing, be signed by the patient and needs to clearly identify the designated recipient and where the information must be sent.

Per existing requirements of the HIPAA Privacy and Security Rules, healthcare providers or health plans sending identifiable health information, per a patient's request, must take steps to verify the identity of the patient prior to sending the information. They must also conduct checks to ensure the correct records are sent and must implement safeguards to protect the information in transit.

Although the Security Rule requires healthcare providers and health plans to implement safeguards for transmitting identifiable health information, patients also have the right to get their copies through unencrypted channels – such as e-mail – if they so choose. Healthcare providers and health plans are required to advise patients of the risk of receiving information through insecure channels; but if the patient opts for the insecure method, he or she has the right to receive the information in this way.

The requirements for Stage 2 Meaningful Use will provide some patients with more timely, on-line access to relevant digital health information. However, these requirements apply only to entities participating in the Meaningful Use program, and those entities are only required to make this access available to a certain percentage of their patients. HIPAA Rules governing PHI access provide the baseline for all providers using digital records and, for some patients, will constitute the only available pathway for obtaining copies of their data.

Designated Record Sets

When individuals exercise their right to access their PHI or obtain a copy of the PHI held by a HIPAA-covered entity, they must be provided with information that is included in one or more designated record sets.

A designated record set is defined in the HIPAA Privacy Rule – 45 CFR 164.501 – as a group of records maintained by or for a covered entity. A designated record set includes the following types of information:

❖ Medical and billing records maintained by or for a healthcare provider

❖ Enrollment, claims adjudication, payment, and case and/or medical management record systems maintained by or for a health plan or

❖ Records that are used, in whole or in part, by or for a covered entity to make decisions about individuals, even if that information has not actually been used to make a decision about the individual who is requesting access.

The term "Record" includes any items, collections, or groupings of information that includes protected health information that is maintained, collected, used, or shared by or on behalf of a covered entity.

Individuals have the right to access the information for as long as it is held by a covered entity or a business associate of a covered entity. That includes information that is stored onsite or offsite, in any form, including PHI that originated from another covered entity.

Charging for Copies of PHI

As previously mentioned, HIPAA covered entities are permitted to impose a fee for responding to requests from individuals who exercise their right to obtain a copy of their health information.

The fees charged must be reasonable and cost-based and can include the cost of creating a summary of health information or providing an explanation – If a summary or explanation has been requested by the patient – the cost of labor for copying information, the cost of supplies such as paper or electronic media if an electronic copy is requested, and postage costs, if the individual has chosen to have the information mailed. HIPAA-covered entities are not permitted to charge for the time it takes to locate, retrieve, and handle PHI.

There are three methods that can be used for calculating fees: Actual costs, average costs, or a flat fee. If the actual cost method is used, an individual should be told in advance approximately how much the fee will be. Average costs can be calculated and a schedule of costs created for different types of request. The cost of any media that is required to satisfy the request can be added to that charge. The flat fee method allows a charge up to a maximum of $6.50, inclusive of all labor, supplies, and postage costs for supplying copies of electronically maintained PHI.

Amendments to Healthcare Records

One of main reasons why patients should be encouraged to obtain a copy of their PHI is to check their records for any errors. If errors are found, a request to amend healthcare records can be submitted in writing. It is acceptable to require a reason for an amendment to be provided as long as the individual is notified in advance. It is also necessary for a covered entity to document the persons or offices responsible for processing these requests.

If the request is accepted, the amendment must be made within 60 days of receiving the amendment request. It is possible to extend this time limit by 30 days provided that the individual is notified in writing and is provided with a valid reason why the delay is necessary. The individual must be notified if the amendment request has been accepted and the covered entity should obtain agreement from the individual if the amendment needs to be shared with others. That information must then be shared within a reasonable time frame.

It is permitted to deny a request to amend health records if the PHI was not created by the covered entity, provided the originator is still able to act on an amendment request. A request can also be denied if the request requires changes to information that is not part of the designated record set, if the record would not be available for inspection or is accurate and complete.

If the request is denied, the individual must be notified of the reason why the request was denied. They must also be informed that they have a right to submit a written statement disagreeing with the denial, be informed that they have the right to include the request and denial in any future disclosures of PHI, and the individual should be told how a complaint can be filed with the HHS. The contact information of an employee of the covered entity responsible for handling complaints should also be provided.

Accounting for Disclosures of PHI

HIPAA-covered entities must create and implement policies and procedures for recording and maintaining a list of disclosures of protected health information, both by the covered entity and their business associates. Disclosures do not need to be recorded if they:

- ❖ Are required for treatment, payment, or healthcare operations
- ❖ Information is disclosed to the patient or their nominated representative

- ❖ Disclosures are made to individuals involved in an individual's healthcare or payment for healthcare
- ❖ If the disclosure is pursuant to an authorization
- ❖ Involves the disclosure of a limited data set
- ❖ Disclosures are made for national security or law enforcement purposes

Individuals have a right to an accounting of disclosures and must be provided, on request, with a list of the recorded disclosures of their PHI for 6 years prior to the date that the request is made. They should be provided with the date and time of access, the name of the person/entity that accessed the information, a description of what the individual/entity did with the information (created, modified, accessed, or deleted information), and a description of the information that was accessed.

The request must be acted on within 60 days of the request being received. It is not permissible to charge an individual for exercising their right to be provided with this information in the first instance in any 12 month period. A reasonable, cost-based fee can be charged for processing any subsequent requests in the same 12-month period.

Notice of Privacy Practices

Any use or disclosure of Protected Health Information for treatment, payment, or healthcare operations must be consistent with the covered entity's Notice of Privacy Practices (NPPs). A covered entity is required to provide patients or plan members with adequate notice of its privacy practices, including the uses or disclosures of the individual's information together with the individual's rights with respect to that information.

The HIPAA Privacy Rule gave individuals a fundamental new right to be informed of the privacy practices of their health plans and of most of their healthcare providers, as well as to be informed of their privacy rights with respect to their personal health information. Health plans and covered healthcare providers are required to develop and distribute a notice that provides a clear explanation of these rights and practices. The notice is intended to focus individuals' attention on privacy issues and concerns, and prompt them to have discussions with their health plans and healthcare providers.

The HIPAA Privacy Rule states that an individual has a right to adequate notice of how a covered entity may use and disclose protected health information, as well as his or her right to privacy, and the covered entity's obligations with respect to any information that is stored. Most covered entities must develop and provide individuals with this notice of their privacy practices, although the HIPAA Privacy Rule does not require the following covered entities to issue NPPs:

❖ Healthcare clearinghouses, if the only protected health information they create or receive is in the capacity of a business associate of another covered entity. – 45 CFR 164.500(b)(1)

- ❖ A correctional institution that is a covered entity (e.g., that has a covered healthcare provider component)

- ❖ A group health plan that does not create or receive PHI other than a summary or enrollment/disenrollment information, if benefits are provided through one or more contracts of insurance HMOs/health insurance issuers – 45 CFR 164.520(a).

Other than the above exceptions, covered entities are required to provide a notice in plain language that describes:

- ❖ How the covered entity may use and disclose an individual's protected health information

- ❖ The individual's rights with respect to PHI and how the individual may exercise those rights, including how the individual may lodge a complaint with the covered entity

- ❖ The covered entity's legal duties with respect to the information held, including a statement that the covered entity is required by law to ensure the privacy of protected health information.

- ❖ The contact details for further information about the covered entity's privacy policies

- ❖ The date that the privacy practices are effective

Providing the Notice

A covered entity must make its notice available to any person who asks for it and make it available on any website it maintains, if that site provides information about its customer services or benefits. In this regard, it is important to make a distinction: A website privacy policy is not the same as a Notice of Privacy Practices (NPP).

Health Plans must also:

- ❖ Provide the notice to individuals already covered by a health plan and to new enrollees at the time of enrollment

- ❖ Provide a revised notice to individuals covered by the plan within 60 days of a material revision

- ❖ Notify individuals covered by the plan of the availability of, and how to obtain, the notice at least once every three years

Covered Direct Treatment Providers must also:

Provide the notice to the individual no later than the date of first service delivery and, except in an emergency treatment situation, make a good faith effort to obtain the individual's written acknowledgment of receipt of the notice. If an acknowledgment cannot be obtained, the provider must document his or her efforts to obtain the acknowledgment and the reason why it was not obtained. In addition, the provider must send an electronic notice automatically and contemporaneously in response to the individual's first request for service.

In an emergency treatment situation, provide the notice after the emergency situation has ended. In these situations, providers are not required to make a good faith effort to obtain a written acknowledgment from individuals.

Make the latest notice (i.e., the one that reflects any changes in privacy policies) available at the provider's office or facility (posted for viewing) for individuals to request and take away with them. A covered entity may email the notice to an individual if the individual agrees to receive an electronic notice.

Organizational Options

Any covered entity, including a hybrid entity or an affiliated covered entity, may choose to develop more than one notice, such as when an entity performs different types of covered functions (i.e., the functions that make it a health plan, a healthcare provider or a healthcare clearinghouse) and there are variations in its privacy practices among these covered functions. Covered entities are encouraged to provide individuals with the most specific notice possible.

Covered entities that participate in an organized healthcare arrangement may choose to produce a single but joint notice if certain requirements are met. For example, the joint notice must describe the covered entities and the service delivery sites to which it applies. If any one of the participating covered entities provides the joint notice to an individual, the notice distribution requirement with respect to that individual is met for all of the covered entities.

An example of a Notice of Privacy Practices can be found on the OCR´s website.

5. The Security Rule

- ❖ The HIPAA Security Rule
- ❖ The Difference between PHI and ePHI
- ❖ Technical Safeguards
- ❖ Physical Safeguards
- ❖ Administrative Safeguards
- ❖ Policies, Sanctions and Training
- ❖ Contingency and Disaster Recovery Plans
- ❖ Risk Analysis and Risk Management

The HIPAA Security Rule

"The HIPAA Security Rule establishes national standards to protect individuals' electronic personal health information that is created, received, used, or maintained by a covered entity. The Security Rule requires appropriate administrative, physical and technical safeguards to ensure the confidentiality, integrity, and security of electronic Protected Health Information".

Definition provided by the US Department of Health and Human Services

Whereas the HIPAA Privacy Rule deals with the integrity of PHI in general, the HIPAA Security Rule deals with electronic protected health information (ePHI) and is a response to the increasing use of personal mobile devices in the workplace.

The professional use of personal mobile devices in the healthcare industry is significant. More than 80 percent of physicians own at least one mobile device (iPhone, Android phone, Blackberry, iPad, tablet or notebooks etc.) with approximately 25 percent utilizing at least two such devices in his or her practice, according to a study on the use of mobile devices in the healthcare industry by Gray Reed & McGraw, P.C

The risk of an unauthorized disclosure of ePHI from a personal mobile device is significant; yet many healthcare organizations have actively pursued "Bring Your Own Device" (BYOD) policies because of the convenience of personal devices, the ease of use and the considerable cost savings in comparison to company-purchased devices. This can all too easily lead to unauthorized disclosures of ePHI, in particular in the following scenarios:

- ❖ The mobile device is misplaced by the user or is lost or stolen, allowing an unauthorized third party to access ePHI

- ❖ The mobile device is left unoccupied or viewable where an unauthorized third party may access it

- ❖ An unauthorized individual "hacks" the mobile device's database or accesses ePHI through an insecure channel of communication

- ❖ Transferring or placing information on a mobile device (or even a flash drive) that is not encrypted

- ❖ The mobile device is traded in without first securely and permanently wiping the data

You may ask yourself "Why would anybody want to access patient healthcare information?" There are in fact many reasons.

Medical records are worth more to hackers than credit cards. With stolen medical records and personal identifiers, hackers can steal identities to obtain loans or credit, get free medical treatment or acquire drugs that can be resold on the black market. Combined with a false provider number, insurance companies can be billed for treatment that has never taken place or for medical equipment that has never been delivered.

Furthermore, medical identity theft is often not immediately identified by a patient or their provider – giving criminals years to milk stolen medical records. That makes medical data considerably more valuable than credit cards, which tend to be quickly canceled by banks once fraud is detected.

So, whereas the original 1996 Healthcare Insurance Portability and Accountability Act was intended to "combat waste, fraud and abuse in health insurance and healthcare delivery", one of the main objectives of the HIPAA Security Rule is to protect individuals from becoming victims of fraud and abuse.

The Difference Between PHI and ePHI

PHI relates to all protected health information irrespective of its format. Electronic "PHI" (ePHI) is classified as all protected health information that is stored, transmitted or used electronically.

Irrespective of whether ePHI is stored on a desktop computer that only has access to an intranet connection or on a personal mobile device, the HIPAA Security Rule guidelines must be implemented whenever ePHI is in transit or at rest. At rest means the device on which ePHI has been saved (computer hard drive, flash drive, personal mobile device) and in transit relates to any electronic communication of that information (text, IMS, email, pager, file transfer, etc.).

The HIPAA Security Rule also covers how ePHI can be accessed, and by whom, and requires administrative, physical and technical safeguards to be developed and implemented to prevent unauthorized data access. That includes addressing common security gaps and vulnerabilities which could be exploited by hackers to gain access to ePHI and to prevent the exposure of ePHI should a device be lost or stolen.

The HIPAA Security Rule ensures patients and their ePHI are protected, as well as healthcare facilities and health insurance providers.

In today´s technological environment, it is essential that all covered entities take notice of the Security Rule to ensure full compliance with HIPAA.

Technical Safeguards

In our "Background and Objectives of HIPAA" we defined the technical safeguards of the HIPAA Security Rule as being there to "protect communications containing PHI when they are transmitted electronically over open networks".

The Security Rule technical safeguards concern the technology and related policies and procedures that protect ePHI and control access to it, and they apply to all forms of ePHI. The HIPAA Security Rule requires a covered entity to comply with the technical safeguards standards; however it does not go as far as to stipulate the exact methods covered entities must use to protect ePHI.

There is some flexibility as to which security measures are implemented to protect data, provided they offer the appropriate degree of protection. That said, a few specific requirements for types of technology to implement are identified in the HIPAA Security Rule.

Together with reasonable and appropriate administrative and physical safeguards, successful implementation of the technical safeguards will help to ensure that a covered entity protects the confidentiality, integrity and availability of ePHI.

What are the HIPAA Technical Safeguards?

The key areas that hospital administrators and practice managers need to be aware of are:

Access Controls – These controls ensure ePHI can only be accessed by authorized users who have been granted access rights. Mechanisms should be implemented that identify and track user activity, automatically log the user out of the system after a period of inactivity and allow access to ePHI during an emergency.

Audit Controls – These are the overall controls that are put in place to monitor, record and examine all ePHI activity. It is recommended that they are configured in such a way that they complement existing EHR mechanisms and can be used to conduct required risk assessments and adjust access controls and staff policies as necessary.

Integrity – Maintaining the integrity of ePHI means implementing controls to ensure that it is not destroyed or altered in a way that is non-compliant with HIPAA. This not only applies to ePHI in transit, but also at rest — which is covered in the physical safeguards.

Person or Entity Authentication – This safeguard is there to ensure that a person who wants access to ePHI is who they say they are. This is usually achieved by passwords or PINs being allocated by an appointed administrator, who has the ability to PIN-lock a device if a risk assessment shows that there is the threat of an ePHI breach such as if a device is lost or stolen.

Transmission Security – The security of ePHI during transmission should be established by the use of data encryption. ePHI should be rendered "unreadable, undecipherable or unusable" so that any healthcare or payment information is of no use to an unauthorized third party. Effective encryption also helps covered entities avoid a substantial fine should a breach of ePHI occur.

Physical Safeguards

The physical safeguards are a set of rules and guidelines outlined in the HIPAA Security Rule that focus on physical access to ePHI and how PHI is stored.

There are four standards in the physical safeguards:

- ❖ Facility Access Controls
- ❖ Workstation Use
- ❖ Workstation Security
- ❖ Devices and Media Controls
- ❖ Facility Access Controls

Facility Access Controls

Facility access controls outline the policies and procedures covered entities must put in place to properly authenticate and authorize access to places where ePHI data is housed. In today's world, this means putting proper procedures in place to ensure that only essential and authorized personnel have access to data centers, server cabinets, storerooms and any other locations where ePHI is stored. This includes IT storerooms where old computer equipment is held. Many digital devices contain stored ePHI, including digital photocopiers, scanners and printers and access to these devices must also be controlled.

The first implementation specification in the facility access controls standards is "Contingency Operations". In short, covered entities should have a plan in place that ensures that in an emergency, the right people have access to the facilities where ePHI is physically housed. Effectively, this means putting together a plan so that in an emergency – a data center outage for example – it is possible for ePHI to be accessed or a backup copy of ePHI to be recovered.

It is also important to make sure there is a way to restore the data elsewhere if needed. The data restoration step is typically part of a disaster recovery plan. For example, if the data center housing a HIPAA compliant application loses power, it has to be possible to restore or bring up the application in a second data center (which is why cloud computing is so popular). The rationale for this implementation specification is pretty straightforward. It ensures that even in an emergency situation, access to a ePHI is not interrupted. Just because a computer system is down, doctors still need access to patient records in a timely manner to ensure the provision of healthcare services is not interrupted.

The second implementation specification is called the Facility Security Plan. As the name implies, covered entities need to implement policies and procedures to properly secure and protect the physical facility where ePHI data is housed. Covered entities should establish plans to reasonably and appropriately prevent unauthorized physical access, tampering and theft of ePHI.

Whether covered entities have an on-site server room, or they host their applications in a shared data center, it is their responsibility to ensure that the facility is properly protected. The protection deployed will depend on many factors, such as the size and type of the covered entity, the volume of data stored and the nature of the data which is held. Protection measures could range from making sure a server room is always locked to adding a digital keypad to the section of the building where the server room is located. It may also be appropriate to employ a private security company to patrol the facility. What is important is that there is a plan in place, that it is documented, and all appropriate personnel are aware of it. The plan must also be regularly tested and verified to be effective.

The third implementation specification is called Access Control and Validation Procedures. This specification calls for covered entities to put procedures in place to ensure that the people accessing the facility where ePHI is housed are indeed who they say they are, and that their access to ePHI is in accordance with his or her role in the organization.

If someone shows up at the location where ePHI is housed claiming to be a computer server technician dispatched to replace a faulty hard drive, the facility procedures must ensure that access to ePHI is not inadvertently provided to an unauthorized person.

The fourth and final implementation specification in the facility access controls standards calls for a covered entity to implement procedures to document any modifications to the facility where ePHI is housed that may affect the facility's security. The procedures put in place should document any additions, changes, removals and repairs to the physical facility housing the ePHI data. Common items logged may include: Replacing a broken digital keypad, upgrading the covered entity's video surveillance system, rekeying server room keys and even the reissue of a security badge to authorized personnel.

Workstation Use

The Workstation Use standard states that covered entities must define what each workstation can be used for, how the work on the workstation is performed and the environment surrounding workstations when they are used to access ePHI.

A workstation, in the eyes of the Department of Health and Human Services, is any electronic device that can be used to access ePHI, which includes desktop computers, laptops, mobile devices (including personal mobile phones that have access to ePHI) and tablets. The definition as it is written in the Security Rule is purposely broad to account for all future devices that have not yet come to the market.

Covered entities have to implement policies and procedures to ensure that ePHI access from electronic devices is secure, which includes defining what workstations can be used for. For example, it is possible to be specific and state that workstations can only be used to access an EHR system or that they can only be used by doctors to record patient medical conditions or for doctor-to-patient communications.

It is also common for covered entities to list what cannot be done on a workstation – such as checking personal emails. When policies are defined for this standard, it is possible to be workstation-specific (e.g., by workstation asset ID) or location-specific (e.g., workstations in building 3) or even by workstation type (e.g., every company issued tablet).

Next, the manner in which work is done on the workstations has to be defined. For example, the patient billing system cannot be used with other software, like a web browser, running in the background. Or each user password for the EHR system must be a minimum of eight alphanumeric characters in length, contain a combination of upper- and lower-case characters and cannot include words found in a dictionary.

Finally, the environment surrounding the workstations has to be defined when they are used to access ePHI. Covered entities can again be very specific and restrict ePHI access to only workstations on the third floor, for example.

Parameters can be set around how data is accessed, such as allowing laptops to be used to access ePHI while off company property as long as they are not connected to the internet via public Wi-Fi and provided that the connection is through a secure VPN. Indeed, when policies relating to workstation use are being defined, keep in mind employees who work in satellite offices or from home. Policies and procedures have to be in place for them as well. Also do not neglect to consider personal mobile devices brought into the workplace or the use of personal devices at home that can potentially be used to access ePHI.

Workstation Security

Workstation Security is closely related to the workstation use standard but there is an important distinction between the two. The workstation use standard addresses the policies and procedures for how workstations should be used, whereas the workstation security standard addresses how workstations are to be physically protected from unauthorized users.

Every covered entity is different, and the Security Rule again calls for reasonable and appropriate measures to be put in place by each entity. In other words, risk assessments should be conducted to determine the level of physical security that is required around each workstation.

Some measures that are easy to implement include ensuring that workstations are positioned in such a way to prevent unauthorized individuals from viewing the screen – by using privacy filters for example – and measures to make it harder for the devices to be improperly accessed. It may also be appropriate for covered entities to place workstations with access to ePHI in locked rooms.

Only by conducting a full and thorough risk assessment is it possible to determine the risks that exist in a particular facility. The results of that assessment can then be used to develop the appropriate controls based on the covered entity´s physical set-up and requirements.

Device and Media Controls

The fourth and final standard in the physical safeguards is Device and Media Controls. This standard calls for covered entities to "implement policies and procedures that govern the receipt and removal of hardware and electronic media that contain electronic protected health information, into and out of a facility, and the movement of these items within the facility."

The definition is a bit long-winded, but this is because in the eyes of the Department of Health and Human Services, electronic media is any medium that can be used to store or transfer ePHI, and this includes: Computer hard drives, removable flash drives, portable USB drives, and DVDs. Technically, an iPad or any other personal mobile device is also considered electronic media since it can be used to store ePHI either directly, when mapped as a portable hard drive, or indirectly using apps like Google Drive or Box.

Disposal

The first required implementation specification is titled Disposal. Covered entities must put in place policies and procedures to "address the final disposition of electronic protected health information, and/or the hardware or electronic media on which it is stored." In other words, when each electronic media device reaches end of life, covered entities must properly process the electronic media and be absolutely sure all ePHI stored on the digital media has been permanently erased.

Bear in mind that digital devices which are not specifically used to store ePHI may also come into contact with protected health information and maintain a record of that information. This includes digital printers, scanners, photocopiers and fax machines. When files are sent to digital printers, they can be stored on internal memory chips and hard drives and these will similarly need to be erased before recycling or returning to a leasing company.

There are several ways to accomplish this. One way is to degauss the electronic media. Degaussing is a process in which a strong magnetic field is applied to magnetic based electronic media such as some computer hard drives which permanently erases the stored content. The degaussing process does not work on newer storage media such as solid-state drives and flash drives which are impervious to magnetic fields. Many academic institutions have looked for ways to effectively erase content on non-magnetic drives and have concluded the only sure method is to completely destroy the media. Covered entities need to carefully take inventory of the electronic media currently in use and come up with steps to properly erase content before disposal.

Media Re-Use

The next required implementation specification is titled Media Re-Use. If covered entities wish to re-use electronic media rather than dispose of them, they are required to put plans in place to ensure all ePHI stored on those devices is permanently destroyed or rendered unreadable before re-use. As pointed out previously, while clearing content on magnetic based storage devices is a fairly easy process, clearing content on non-magnetic storage devices is much more difficult.

For example, deleting files from a desktop computer and emptying the recycle bin is not sufficient as even deleted data can be restored or reconstructed. So once again, a careful review of the electronic media currently used by covered entities should be conducted and procedures developed to ensure that all data is permanently erased.

Accountability

Accountability is the next implementation specification. This implementation specification calls for covered entities to keep records of the movement of hardware and electronic media used to access or store ePHI and to log the person accountable for the move. Covered entities have the flexibility to decide what is considered to be reasonable and appropriate record keeping. Ideally, if a server is removed from the server room for servicing or if a faulty hard drive is replaced for example, covered entities should log the specific device involved and the person who has authorized the change.

Data Backup and Storage

The last implementation specification is Data Backup and Storage. Before any hardware and electronic media are physically moved, a backup of the ePHI contained on each media device must be made. This ensures if anything were to happen to the hardware during a move, such as damage, loss or theft, the contained ePHI is protected and data loss is prevented. Given the rise in the use of ransomware, backups are more important than ever. Multiple copies of ePHI should be made and at least one copy should be stored securely off site.

Preventing Data Breaches

Data Encryption	Encrypt all protected data to prevent unauthorized access
Compliant Cloud Storage	Use verified secure, encrypted off-site storage for protected data
Secure Messaging	Use verified secure, encrypted internal communications system
Software Updates	Install all patches and updates promptly
Virus and Malware Control	Maintain anti-virus and malware software; scan regularly
Staff Training	Train all employees on compliance obligations and procedures
Secure Disposal	Shred or hire a document disposal service; erase and reformat electronic media
Business Associates	Verify compliance by all business associates

Administrative Safeguards

Administrative safeguards are actions, policies and procedures which manage the selection, development, implementation and maintenance of security measures that safeguard electronic protected health information. Administrative safeguards also help HIPAA-covered entities to manage the conduct of their – and their business associate's – workforce in relation to the protection of that information.

Administrative safeguards encompass more than half of HIPAA Security Rule requirements. Like the technical and physical safeguards, many of these items are not mandatory but "addressable". This means that all covered entities must give full consideration to each point and assess the relevance of that measure to their own organization. If it is not appropriate to implement a particular (addressable) safeguard – or if it is possible to implement alternative safeguards that offer a similar or greater degree of protection – this is permissible.

Having administrative safeguards in place, in combination with other safeguards, makes it easier for security officers to prevent ePHI data breaches and it also allows them to take rapid action when data is compromised or is otherwise exposed.

The Security Rule states that administrative safeguards are, "administrative actions, and policies and procedures, to manage the selection, development, implementation, and maintenance of security measures to protect ePHI and to manage the conduct of the covered entity's workforce in relation to the protection of that information."

This basically calls for those responsible for security in healthcare organizations to evaluate preexisting security controls, to accurately and thoroughly analyze risks and to document solutions and translate these into policies and procedures.

The standards for the administrative safeguards consist of:

- ❖ The Security Management Process
- ❖ Assigned Security Responsibility
- ❖ Workforce Security
- ❖ Information Access Management
- ❖ Security Awareness and Training
- ❖ Security Incident Procedures
- ❖ Contingency Planning
- ❖ Evaluation
- ❖ Business Associate Contracts and Other Arrangements

The Security Management Process

The Security Management Process covers the implementation of policies and procedures to prevent, detect, contain and correct security violations.

These are categorized into 4 implementation specifications:

Risk Analysis (Required)

A risk analysis is one of the most important elements of the HIPAA Security Rule, yet it is one of the most common areas of noncompliance, as was highlighted by both the pilot and second phase HIPAA audit programs. A risk analysis is a procedure by which the entire organization is assessed for potential security vulnerabilities and risks to the confidentiality, integrity and availability of electronic protected health information (ePHI) held by the covered entity.

If a risk analysis is conducted that is not comprehensive – I.e. does not cover all aspects of data security for both physical PHI and ePHI – security vulnerabilities are likely to remain that could place the confidentiality of health records in jeopardy. Only by identifying ALL risks can an organization take action to effectively manage those risks.

A risk analysis is not a onetime action, but a continuous process of reevaluation and assessment that should take place at regular intervals, in particular after a material change in HIPAA legislation or as part of the process of implementing new software or computer systems that have potential to come into contact with PHI.

An incomplete or non-compliant risk analysis is one of the most common HIPAA violations uncovered by OCR when investigating complaints, data breaches and preforming compliance audits. Due to these failures and the importance of the risk assessment, OCR has released guidance on this vital implementation specification. The guidance and required risk analysis tool can be downloaded from the OCR website. The risk analysis is available as either a written questionnaire or a software tool.

The risk analysis should not be confused with a gap analysis. A gap analysis is a partial assessment which provides a high-level overview of controls that have been put in place to secure electronic protected health information and identify any areas where gaps may exist.

The gap analysis can be conducted to review compliance with certain implementation specifications of the HIPAA Security Rule and is defined by OCR as "a narrowed examination of a covered entity or business associate's enterprise to assess whether certain controls or safeguards required by the Security Rule have been implemented." HIPAA-covered entities are encouraged to perform a gap analysis.

A gap analysis is not a substitute for a risk analysis, which is much more in depth and applies to all risks to all ePHI created, received, maintained, or transmitted by a HIPAA-covered entity.

Risk Management (Required)

Once a risk analysis has been conducted and all potential security vulnerabilities have been identified, the covered entity must then implement security measures sufficient to reduce those risks and vulnerabilities to a reasonable and appropriate level.

Sanction Policy (Required)

A sanction policy must be put in place to allow the covered entity to take action against workforce members who fail to comply with the security policies and procedures of the covered entity. The staff should be made aware of the HIPAA Privacy and Security Rules and must agree to abide by them. All sanctions that will be applied following a violation of HIPAA Rules, such the termination of an employment contract, must be communicated to the staff.

Information System Activity Review (Required)

It is essential that all covered entities implement a system, preferably automated, which logs all system activity relating to ePHI, in particular any requests to access patient records or make amendments to PHI. Audit logs must be created, and the system must be capable of generating security incident tracking reports.

Even the most robust security systems cannot prevent authorized users from accessing ePHI improperly, so it is essential that all attempts to view or alter ePHI are logged, and that these logs are regularly checked for inappropriate access. Inappropriate access is one of the main causes of HIPAA breaches, such as employees snooping on medical records and data theft by authorized users.

Assigned Security Responsibility

A HIPAA security officer should be appointed and given responsibility for the development and implementation of HIPAA policies and procedures relating to data security.

While one person must be given overall responsibility for all security responsibilities, other individuals can be assigned individual responsibilities such as network security, device management or site security, provided they report to the security officer with overall responsibility for HIPAA compliance. In large organizations, it may be necessary to assign tasks to numerous individuals and may be of benefit to appoint separate Privacy and Security officers.

Workforce Security

Access to ePHI must be restricted and carefully controlled, yet healthcare professionals do require access to ePHI in order to do their jobs and provide healthcare services to patients. This means that policies and procedures must be developed to ensure that all members of the workforce have appropriate access to ePHI, as required under the Information Access Management standard, while others must be prevented from viewing ePHI.

Workforce security comprises three implementation specifications:

Authorization and/or Supervision (Addressable)

Policies must be developed and procedures implemented which allow users to be granted authorization to access or amend ePHI commensurate with their position. In practice this means assessing job descriptions to determine what degree of access is required. All members of staff granted access to ePHI must be supervised in locations where data may be accessed.

Workforce Clearance Procedure (Addressable)

A clearance procedure must exist that assesses whether the level of access to ePHI that an individual workforce member needs to perform his or her duties is appropriate. A clearance procedure must verify that an individual has an appropriate level of access to perform their duties.

Termination
Procedures (Addressable)

Just as procedures must be developed to grant users access to essential ePHI, procedures must also be in place to terminate those access rights when they are no longer required, such as following a change in the individual's duties or after the termination of an employment contract.

Information Access Management

The fourth standard covers the management of access to ePHI by members of the workforce who need to view, amend or update ePHI as part of their daily duties. Controlling access is an essential element of data security that limits the potential for accidental or deliberate disclosure of PHI to non-authorized individuals, while also limiting the possibility of erasure or alteration of ePHI.

Information Access Management includes three implementation specifications:

Isolating Healthcare Clearinghouse
Functions (Required)

If a healthcare clearinghouse is part of a larger organization, the clearinghouse must implement policies and procedures that protect the ePHI of the clearinghouse from unauthorized access by the larger organization.

Access Authorization (Addressable)

This specification is similar to that stated in the Workforce Security section, but instead of determining access rights, Access Authorization requires policies and procedures to be implemented for granting access to ePHI, such as through a particular workstation or for specific transactions, programs, processes or other mechanisms.

Access Establishment and Modification (Addressable)

A covered entity must implement policies and procedures that, based upon the entity's access authorization policies, establish, document, review and modify a user's right of access to a workstation, transaction, program, or process.

Security Awareness and Training

One of the most important elements of the administrative safeguards is the provision of training on the HIPAA Security and Privacy Rules, not only for the staff that is granted access to ePHI or may otherwise come into contact with it, but all members of the workforce, including management. Even the most robust security policies can be easily compromised due to poor or non-existent staff training.

In addition to providing training on HIPAA Rules, all employees should be provided with cybersecurity training to teach best practices and alert them to the methods used by cybercriminals to gain access to ePHI, such as phishing, business email compromise, and social engineering. All employees should receive training on how to identify phishing emails and that training must be documented.

Security Awareness and Training includes four implementation specifications:

Security Reminders (Addressable)

The provision of training ensures that the workforce is fully aware of the HIPAA Privacy and Security Rules; however, policies frequently need to be updated and these changes must be communicated to the staff. It is also important to provide the workforce with reminders on the importance of data security and PHI policies and procedures.

All reminders must be documented and a record maintained, while the procedures must govern the issuing of reminders, such as via electronic bulletins, the posting of security reminders on notice boards and the creation of agendas for periodic staff meetings etc.

Protection from Malicious Software (Addressable)

Covered entities must put procedures into place which guard against, detect and report malicious software, including computer viruses such as Trojans, worms, keyloggers, malware, and ransomware. Viruses and malware can be used by external parties to gain access to data or to convince authorized personnel to divulge their login credentials and security keys. Both ransomware and malware can also damage, delete or otherwise alter data. See the Contingency Planning section for more information.

All members of the workforce must receive training to help them identify potentially dangerous software and training and staff should be aware of how, and to whom, they should report the potential installation of malicious software. This includes developing policies which restrict how the internet is used and what can be downloaded.

Log-in Monitoring (Addressable)

Procedures must be developed for monitoring log-in attempts and reporting discrepancies. A system must be in place that can log access attempts, such as multiple attempts to gain access to ePHI using incorrect passwords or usernames. Systems can be configured to log these attempts and generate security reports or alerts, or even to block access for a particular user or device. One measure which can be employed is the blocking of a login after a set number of access attempts have failed – termed rate limiting.

Password Management (Addressable)

Procedures must be developed to cover creating, changing and safeguarding passwords used to access ePHI. If passwords are not automatically assigned, training must be provided on creating secure passwords, such as not using dates of birth, children's names, dictionary words or any commonly used insecure passwords that can easily be guessed (password, 12345678, etc.).

Policies should be developed that require users to change their passwords at regular intervals and employees should be advised about how passwords can be safeguarded. Best practices for passwords often change. The effectiveness of forced password resets every 3 months has been questioned, as has the use of random strings of digits, letters, and symbols as these often have to be written down in order to be remembered. Covered entities should consult the guidance issued by NIST on passwords and best practices – See NIST Special Publication 800-63B for further information and keep abreast of changes to access control recommendations.

Security Incident Procedures

Even the most security conscious healthcare organizations that have implemented multi-layered security defenses and are fully HIPAA-compliant will, at some point in time, experience a security incident. While it is possible to reduce and manage risk, it is not possible to eliminate it entirely. Covered entities must therefore implement procedures that allow these incidents to be reported quickly, and to the appropriate personnel.

There is only one implementation specification:

Response and Reporting (Required)

This specification states that all HIPAA-covered entities must be able to "identify and respond to suspected or known security incidents; mitigate, to the extent practicable, harmful effects of security incidents that are known to the covered entity; and document security incidents and their outcomes."

There are numerous types of security incident, and the workforce must be aware how to "identify and respond to suspected or known security incidents; mitigate, to the extent practicable, harmful effects of security incidents that are known to the covered entity; and document security incidents and their outcomes."

Examples of security incidents include, but are not limited to:

❖ Loss or theft of portable devices containing unencrypted ePHI

❖ Stolen or divulged passwords

❖ Potential phishing attacks and suspicious emails

❖ Computer viruses and malware

❖ Corrupted backup tapes that do not allow ePHI to be restored

❖ Break-ins resulting in the theft of devices containing ePHI

❖ The use of old logins – such as those of terminated members of staff – to access ePHI

❖ The accessing of ePHI by non-authorized members of staff

Procedures must be developed which allow a rapid and adequate response to each of these threats, and any others that may exist in a particular organization.

Contingency Planning

Access to ePHI must be maintained at all times, even during emergencies. Procedures must therefore be developed to ensure that this is the case. Covered entities must "Establish (and implement as needed) policies and procedures for responding to an emergency or other occurrence (for example, fire, vandalism, system failure, and natural disaster) that damages systems that contain ePHI."

Contingency Planning includes five implementation specifications:

Data Backup Plan (Required)

Entities must establish and implement procedures to create and maintain retrievable exact copies of ePHI. All data, including health information, diagnostic images, medical records, accounting information and other electronic documents must be frequently backed up, and any physical backup tapes, if used, must be stored off-site in a secure location protected by the physical safeguards mentioned above.

Backup are one of the most important defenses against ransomware attacks which encrypt ePHI to prevent access. Without a backup, data may not be able to be recovered. Even payment of a ransom is no guarantee that valid keys will be supplied to unlock files encrypted by ransomware. Ransomware can also encrypt backup copies of ePHI and delete Windows Shadow Copies. At least one copy of ePHI should therefore be stored on an air-gapped device – I.e. one which is not connected to the network or internet.

Disaster Recovery Plan (Required)

HIPAA-covered entities must establish and implement procedures to restore any loss of data and this plan must be reviewed and revised frequently and tested.

Emergency Mode Operation Plan (Required)

Even during a power outage or other emergency situation such as a server malfunction, procedures must exist to ensure the continuation of critical business processes and the protection of ePHI while operating in emergency mode.

Testing and Revision Procedures (Addressable)

All Contingency Plan implementation specifications must be subjected to tests to ensure that data can be restored, and emergency operational procedures must similarly be subjected to live tests to ensure they are effective. These tests should be conducted on a regular basis and policies and procedures revised as appropriate.

Applications and Data Criticality Analysis (Addressable)

Covered entities are required to "Assess the relative criticality specific applications and data in support of other contingency plan components." This means that all software and computer systems

must be evaluated and given priority for backups –
and restoration of data from backup tapes and
devices – based on their importance to the running
of the organization and the provision of patient
healthcare services.

Evaluation

This standard covers the monitoring and
evaluation of all security measures to ensure that
they continue to offer the appropriate level of
protection to keep ePHI secure.

Over time, systems and personnel will change,
new technology will be introduced, and operational
environments are also subject to change. Naturally,
policies and procedures must be updated to take
these new occurrences and changes into account.

There are no implementation specifications under
this standard. Covered entities are just required to
"Perform a periodic technical and nontechnical
evaluation, based initially upon the standards
implemented under this rule and subsequently, in
response to environmental or operations changes
affecting the security of ePHI that establishes the
extent to which an entity's security policies and
procedures meet the requirements of this subpart
[the Security Rule]."

Business Associate Agreements and Other Arrangements

The last standard under administrative safeguards covers business associates – and their subcontractors. A covered entity is required to enter into a Business Associate Agreement with any third party that creates, receives, maintains, transmits, or otherwise comes into contact with ePHI.

This is a required element, and a covered entity, in accordance with § 164.306 [the Security Standards: General Rules], may permit a business associate to create, receive, maintain, or transmit ePHI on the covered entity's behalf only if the covered entity obtains satisfactory assurances, in accordance with § 164.314(a) [the Organizational Requirements] that the business associate will appropriately safeguard the information."

There is a single implementation specification for this standard:

Written contracts

Covered entities must "Document the satisfactory assurances required by paragraph (b) (1) [the Business Associate Contracts and Other Arrangements] of this section through a written contract or other arrangement with the business associate that meets the applicable requirements of §164.314(a) [the Organizational Requirements]."

6. The Breach Notification Rule – What to do in the Event of a Breach

- ❖ The HIPAA Breach Notification Rule
- ❖ OCR Settlements and Civil Monetary Penalties

The HIPAA Breach Notification Rule

Even with all the safeguards in the world, patient healthcare and payment information can be compromised. Risks can be effectively managed, but it is impossible to prevent employees snooping or to prevent human error entirely. As mentioned in our explanation of the Security Rule, mobile devices can be misplaced, left unattended, be stolen or traded in without proper data removal, and even with multi-layered defenses, cyberattacks can still occur.

If covered entities follow the administrative, technical and physical safeguards of the HIPAA Security Rule – and ePHI is encrypted to a standard that would make it "unusable, indecipherable or unreadable" – it may not be necessary to report data breaches. Data breaches only need to be reported when there is a breach of unsecured (non-encrypted) ePHI.

The definition of a breach provided by the US Department of Health and Human Services is as follows:

"A breach is, generally, an impermissible use or disclosure under the Privacy Rule that compromises the security or privacy of the Protected Health Information." An impermissible use or disclosure of protected health information is presumed to be a breach unless the covered entity or business associate, as applicable, demonstrates that there is a low probability that the protected health information has been compromised based on a risk assessment that includes at least the following factors:

❖ The nature and extent of the protected health information involved, including the types of identifiers and the likelihood of re-identification

❖ The unauthorized person who used or accessed the protected health information or to whom any disclosure has been made

❖ Whether the protected health information was actually acquired or viewed

❖ The extent to which the risk to the protected health information has been mitigated

If, despite all precautions, a breach has occurred which potentially could result in the unauthorized disclosure of a patient´s healthcare and/or payment information, the affected patients must be informed within 60 days of the discovery of the breach. The Secretary of the Department of Health and Human Services must also be notified, by submitting a breach summary through the Office for Civil Rights breach portal.

Informing a Patient of a Breach of ePHI

To inform a patient of a breach of PHI or ePHI, a notification must be sent by first class mail to the last known address of the patient, the next of kin if the patient is deceased or the parent or guardian of a child under the age of eighteen whose healthcare information has been compromised.

If the breach requires urgent attention because of possible imminent misuse of PHI, the patient should also be contacted by telephone or by any other means of communication that is considered appropriate. The content of the notification should include:

❖ A brief description of what happened, including the date of the breach and the date of discovery of the breach

❖ A description of the types of information that were compromised in the breach (personal identifiers such as name, address, Social Security number, account numbers, etc.)

❖ The measures individuals should take to protect themselves from potential harm

❖ A brief description of what the covered entity is doing to investigate the breach, to mitigate harm, and prevent a repeat of the breach

❖ Contact details for individuals to ask questions or request further information, which should include a toll-free number, an email address, website or postal address

Informing the Department of Health and Human Services

Informing the Department of Health and Human Services that a breach of PHI has occurred is done using the department´s online notification form. The procedures for reporting a breach of PHI differ depending on the number of patient records that have been compromised (or have potentially been compromised):

Data Breaches Affecting Fewer Than 500 Individuals

If a breach of unsecured protected health information affects fewer than 500 individuals, a covered entity must notify the Secretary of the breach within 60 days of the end of the calendar year in which the breach was discovered.

This does not mean that a covered entity must wait until the end of the calendar year to report breaches affecting fewer than 500 individuals. As a "Best Practice" it is advisable to report the breach as soon as the details of the breach are known.

A covered entity may report all of its breaches affecting fewer than 500 individuals on one date, but a separate notice must be issued for each breach incident.

In early 2015, OCR updated the breach reporting portal and replaced the online form with a JavaScript wizard to guide the user through the reporting process. This new system streamlines the collection of data, allows specific questions to be asked and ensures that all information relating to the breach is recorded in sufficient detail. Compliance officers should familiarize themselves with the data that must be entered after a breach, rather than leaving the reporting until the year end when it may be more difficult to obtain the necessary information.

While the Secretary of the Department of Health and Human Services is happy to wait to find out about these smaller breaches, the individuals affected by the breach must still be notified within 60 days of the discovery of the breach.

Data Breaches Affecting More Than 500 Individuals

If a breach of unsecured protected health information affects 500 or more individuals, a covered entity must notify the Secretary about the breach without unreasonable delay, and in no case later than 60 calendar days from the discovery of the breach.

If the number of individuals affected by a breach is unknown, the covered entity should provide an estimate and amend the breach report at a later date when more information is known. This can be done by checking the appropriate box to indicate that an addendum to the initial report has been added, making sure the transaction number of the initial breach report is included to ensure the data can be matched up.

Breaches of 500 or more healthcare records also require a substitute breach notice to be uploaded to the website of the covered entity, which should be linked from the home page of the site using prominent link.

A notice about the data breach should also be submitted to a prominent media agency serving the area or region affected by the breach.

Data Breaches Caused by a Business Associate

A business associate of a covered entity that accesses, maintains, retains, modifies, records, stores, destroys, or otherwise holds, uses, or discloses unsecured protected health information shall, following the discovery of a breach of such information, notify the covered entity as soon as possible. The notice must identify each individual whose unsecured protected health information has been, or is reasonably believed to have been, accessed, acquired or disclosed as a result of the breach.

For the purposes of clarification, the HIPAA Breach Notification Rule and the HITECH Notification Rule are practically the same. The notification procedures were established by HITECH in 2009, but slight changes to the definition of breaches were made in the Omnibus Final Rule of 2013.

A more significant change introduced with the Omnibus Final Rule of 2013 was to place the burden of proof on the covered entity, which must determine (through a risk assessment) that a breach of ePHI has not occurred. Previously the onus was on the Office for Civil Rights to prove that a HIPAA breach had occurred, whereas now any potential exposure of PHI is considered to be a breach unless the covered entity can prove otherwise.

OCR Fines and Civil Action

Later in our HIPAA Compliance Guide we discuss how HIPAA is enforced and what happens after the Department of Health and Human Services' Office for Civil Rights has been notified of a breach; however, this is a suitable point to discuss the fines that can be issued by the Office for Civil Rights, and other penalties that can be applied following a breach of PHI or ePHI.

The HIPAA Enforcement Rule is the area of legislation that governs the investigations that follow a breach of PHI, the penalties that can be imposed on covered entities for an avoidable breach and the procedures for hearings.

Covered entities should be aware that the financial penalties that can be issued are based on the efforts that have been made to protect the integrity of patient´s healthcare and payment information prior to the breach, and also the actions taken after the breach to mitigate any damage caused.

HIPAA Breach Financial Penalty Structure

Fines are imposed per violation category and reflect the number of records exposed in a breach, the risk to individuals from the exposure of their data, the severity of the violation, knowledge of the violation, and also the means of the covered entity to cover a fine.

Penalties can easily reach the maximum fine of $1,500,000 per violation category, per calendar year. It should also be noted that the penalties for willful neglect can also lead to criminal charges being filed.

As a point of interest, historic civil cases have shown covered entities to be treated more leniently when they have made an effort to comply with HIPAA and promptly address the breach, take steps to ensure any HIPAA violations are corrected, and measures are introduced to prevent further breaches.

Major Data Breaches in 2018

Type of Breach	Number of Incidents	Percentage of Total Incidents
Theft	42	11%
Hacking or IT Incident	161	44%
Unauthorized or Improper Access/Disclosure	145	39%
Loss	13	4%
Improper Disposal	9	2%

Location of Data Subject to Breach

Location of Data Breach	Number of Incidents	Percentage of Total Incidents
Paper or Film	81	19%
Network Servers	74	18%
Emails	122	29%
Desktop Computers	34	8%
Laptop Computers	27	6%
Electronic Medical/Patient Records	27	7%
Other Electronic Devices	21	6%
Other	35	8%

7. The HIPAA Enforcement Rule – How is HIPAA Compliance Enforced?

How the OCR Regulates HIPAA Privacy, Security & Breach Notification Rules

OCR is responsible for enforcing compliance with the HIPAA Privacy, Security, and Breach Notification Rules. One of the ways that OCR carries out this responsibility is to investigate complaints that have been filed against organizations. OCR may also conduct compliance reviews to determine if covered entities have implemented the appropriate policies and procedures demanded by HIPAA.

OCR also issues guidance and performs education and outreach programs to foster compliance with all requirements of the HIPAA Rules.

However, OCR may only take action over certain types of complaints. The OCR website provides details of what OCR considers during intake and review of a complaint and a description of the types of cases in which it cannot commence enforcement actions.

If OCR accepts a complaint for investigation, it will notify the person who filed the complaint and the covered entity named in it. The complainant and the covered entity are then asked to present information about the incident or problem described in the complaint. OCR may request specific information from each party to gain an understanding of the facts of each case. Covered entities are required by law to cooperate fully with all complaint investigations.

If a complaint describes an action that could be a violation of the criminal provision of HIPAA (42 U.S.C. 1320d-6), OCR may refer the complaint to the Department of Justice for further investigation.

In addition to complaints, OCR investigates all breaches of 500 or more records that are reported through the OCR breach portal to determine whether the breach was the result of noncompliance with HIPAA Rules and whether, through HIPAA compliance, the breach could have been prevented. If some evidence of noncompliance is discovered, a more comprehensive compliance review may be initiated.

OCR reviews all information, or evidence, that it gathers in each case. In some cases, it may determine that the covered entity did not violate the requirements HIPAA. If the evidence indicates that the covered entity was not in compliance, OCR will attempt to resolve the case with the covered entity through:

- ❖ Voluntary compliance;
- ❖ Corrective action; and/or
- ❖ A resolution agreement

Most Privacy and Security Rule investigations are concluded to the satisfaction of OCR through these types of resolutions. OCR notifies the person who filed the complaint and covered entity of the resolution result in writing.

If the covered entity does not take action to resolve the matter in a way that is deemed to be satisfactory, OCR may decide to impose civil money penalties (CMPs) on the covered entity. If CMPs are imposed, the covered entity may request a hearing in which an HHS administrative law judge decides if the penalties are appropriate and are supported by the evidence. Complainants do not receive a portion of CMPs collected from covered entities; instead the penalties are deposited in the U.S. Treasury.

HIPAA Violation Penalties

	TIER 1	TIER 2	TIER 3	TIER 4
Standard Applied	Unaware of violation and by reasonable due diligence would not have known rules were violated	Knew or should have known about violation by exercise of reasonable due diligence	Willful neglect of HIPAA Rules with correction of violation within 30 days of discovery	Willful neglect of HIPAA Rules with no effort to correct violation within 30 days of discovery
Fine per Violation	$100 — $50,000	$1000 — $50,000	$10,000 — $50,000	$50,000
Maximum Fine per Year	$25,000	$100,000	$250,000	$1.5 Million

Background to the OCR Privacy, Security and Breach Notification Pilot Audit Program

The use of health information technology continues to expand in healthcare. New technologies provide many benefits for consumers, but they also introduce new risks to consumer privacy.

The Health Insurance Portability and Accountability Act (HIPAA) and the Health Information Technology for Economic and Clinical Health Act (HITECH) set national minimum standards to protect PHI and effectively manage those risks, such as securing ePHI and issuing breach notifications to individuals affected by data breaches to allow them to take action to protect themselves against identity theft and medical fraud.

HITECH also places a requirement on the HHS – via its Office for Civil Rights – to perform periodic audits of covered entities – including business associates – to assess for compliance with the HIPAA Privacy, Security and Breach Notification Rules.

In 2011, the OCR developed a program of pilot audits to assess the general state of compliance with HIPAA in the healthcare industry, which included an assessment of the controls and processes covered entities have put in place to comply with HIPAA Rules.

HIPAA Compliance Audits

The OCR developed a protocol, or set of instructions, which it then used to measure the efforts of 115 covered entities. As part of OCR's continued commitment to protect health information, the agency instituted a formal evaluation of the effectiveness of its pilot audit program.

The OCR HIPAA audit program analyzed processes, controls and policies of randomly selected covered entities pursuant to the HITECH Act audit mandate. The entire audit protocol was organized around modules, representing the separate elements of patient privacy, data security and the issuing of breach notifications. The combination of these multiple requirements was then tailored to the type of covered entity selected for audit.

The audit protocol covered Privacy Rule requirements for (1) Notice of Privacy Practices relating to PHI, (2) Rights to request privacy protection for PHI, (3) Individuals' access to their PHI, (4) Administrative requirements, (5) Uses and disclosures of PHI, (6) Amendment of PHI, and (7) Accounting of disclosures.

The protocol covered Security Rule requirements for administrative, physical, and technical safeguards, Breach Notification Rule requirements and patient access to their healthcare data. The protocol was made available for public review, although since the pilot audit program was completed, the audit protocol has been amended. Details are available on the HHS website.

Second Round of HIPAA Compliance Audits

The pilot HIPAA audits allowed OCR to gauge HIPAA compliance in healthcare and did not result in fines being issued. The main aim of the audits was to assess compliance to guide future OCR guidance. The second round of HIPAA compliance audits was penciled for late 2014 but suffered many delays and did not start until 2017.

The criteria for the second round differed from the broad nature of the pilot compliance audits. OCR took the information gained from its first round of 115 audits and developed an audit protocol which specifically tested those areas of the HIPAA Privacy, Security and Breach Notification Rules which proved problematic for healthcare organizations, health plans and healthcare clearinghouses. The second round of audits were much narrower in focus and involved many more compliance audits.

OCR announced it will be conducting 400 compliance audits in the second round, involving 350 covered entities and 50 of their business associates.

100 covered entities were selected for a Privacy Rule audit, a further 100 for a Breach Notification Rule audit and 150 for a Security Rule audit. The audits were a mixture of desk-based documentation reviews and compliance audits including a site visit and full paperwork inspection. Financial penalties could be issued for compliance failures identified during the audits, although it is

likely to be some time before any fines are announced.

Enforcement Has Already Begun

The Department of Health and Human Services tasked OCR with policing HIPAA on December 28, 2000 – the date of the issuing of the Privacy Rule. The compliance deadline was April 14, 2003, although it took five years before OCR issued its first fine for noncompliance in 2008. Up until that point over 33,000 HIPAA complaints had been filed with OCR, of which 8,000 were investigated, but no financial penalties had been issued.

The first OCR settlement was reached with Providence Health Services for $100,000 after the loss of backup tapes containing PHI potentially exposed the health information of 386,000 patients. In 2009, further fines were issued, including a $2.25 million fine for CVS Pharmacy Inc., for the improper disposal of patient health records.

In 2010, fines were issued to the Rite Aid Corporation for $1 million, again for improper disposal of health records, a $35,000 fine was issued to Management Services Organization Washington Inc. for an improper disclosure of PHI and in 2011, OCR issued the first fine for denying patients access to their health records. Cignet Health (Prince Georges County, MD) paid a $4.3 million penalty to settle the case.

Since then, OCR has increased its enforcement activities and commonly agrees to 6-figure settlements with HIPAA covered entities and their business associates. Even government departments are not exempt from financial penalties. In July 2011, the loss of a storage device by the Alaska Department of Health and Human Services (DHHS) resulted in a financial penalty of $1.7 million.

In March 2012, OCR reached a settlement with Blue Cross Blue Shield of Tennessee (BCBST) – the first self-reported breach to attract a financial penalty.

In 2014, OCR issued its largest ever fine, resulting in a settlement with New York Presbyterian Hospital and Columbia University for $4.8 million. The breach was caused by the lack of a functioning firewall that resulted in a breach that exposed over 1 million patient health records.

The record was broken again in 2016 with a $5.55 million penalty for Advocate Health network over the theft of desktop computers, laptop computers, and improper PHI access by a business associate. Memorial Healthcare System agreed to settle its case with OCR for $5.5 million in 2017 over insufficient ePHI access controls.

The record was totally smashed in 2018 with a $16 million settlement with Anthem Inc., to resolve multiple HIPAA violations that contributed to the breach of 78.8 million records in 2015. 2018 also saw record financial penalties issued, which totaled $28.7 million.

It may have taken a long time for the first fines to be issued, but now they are coming thick and fast and HIPAA is being policed much more rigorously. Attorneys General are also permitted to take action over HIPAA violations and assist OCR with HIPAA enforcement. Many have now issued fines for violations of HIPAA Rules. The days of lax enforcement of HIPAA Privacy and Security Rules have certainly long since passed.

2018 HIPAA Violation Penalties

Noncompliance fines imposed in 2018: $28,683,400

Anthem,Inc.	**$16,000,000**	**Multiple Violations**
Univ. of Texas, M.D. Anderson Cancer Center	**$4,348,000**	**Disclosure of ePHI/lack of encryption**
Fresenius Medical Care of North America	**$3,500,000**	**Multiple Violations**
Cottage Health	**$3,000,000**	**Unsecured server accessible via internet**
Massachusetts General Hospital	**$515,000**	**Filming patients without consent**
Advanced Care Hospitalists	**$500,000**	**No compliance efforts prior to April 1, 2014**
Brigham & Women's Hospital	**$384,000**	**Filming patients without consent**
Allergy Associates of Hartford	**$125,000**	**Disclosure of PHI to reporter**
Pagosa Springs Medical Center	**$111,400**	**Failure to terminate employee ePHI access**
Boston Medical Center	**$100,000**	**Filming patients without consent**
Filefax, Inc.	**$100,000**	**Improper disclosure of PHI**

8. Secure Communications and HIPAA Compliance

HIPAA-Compliant IT Systems and Electronic Communications

At the heart of HIPAA is the requirement to protect ePHI and to keep all healthcare data private and confidential. While the Health Insurance and Portability and Accountability Act makes numerous recommendations, it is up to covered entities to decide how ePHI is protected.

All IT systems, devices and software that are capable of touching ePHI must be subject to a full risk analysis to ensure that no security vulnerabilities exist which could be exploited to expose the protected health information of patients and health plan members.

Website Security

Doctors and other medical professionals now face increasing pressure to get their businesses online, make use of electronic prescriptions, take web appointments, provide virtual consultations and deliver remote healthcare services. Electronic transactions, websites and patient portals improve the patient experience and are critical for building and sustaining revenue streams in the tightening medical market.

HIPAA Rules require covered entities to ensure that ePHI is protected and secured at all times. All websites, old and new, must therefore be properly designed to ensure that data is secured, or site owners face potential fines that could run into millions of dollars.

So, how can HIPAA Rules be followed in an online environment and how does the legislation apply to websites and online patient portals?

What are the HIPAA Requirements for a Website?

HIPAA is an unusual law in that it makes a lot of recommendations – addressable items – and a few assertions – required items – but in the end it is up to each organization to determine for themselves what they need to do to become compliant. This allows a great deal of flexibility and also creates a great deal of uncertainty. In general, to be HIPAA-compliant, a website must, at a minimum, ensure that all protected health information (ePHI) is safeguarded:

- ❖ Transport Encryption: Data must be encrypted if it is transmitted over the Internet

- ❖ Backup: Data cannot be lost, I.e. it should be backed up and must be recoverable

- ❖ Authorization: Data can only be accessed by authorized personnel using unique credentials

- ❖ Integrity: Data cannot be tampered with or altered

- ❖ Storage Encryption: Data should be encrypted when it is stored or archived

- ❖ Disposal: Data must be permanently erased when it is no longer needed

- ❖ Sharing: If data is located on the web servers of a third party, that entity must agree to comply with HIPAA regulations and a signed HIPAA business associate agreement must be obtained

Does a Simple Website Meet HIPAA Compliance Requirements?

By a simple website, we refer to one set up with any of the popular hosting providers (e.g. GoDaddy) and written using off the shelf software (WordPress for example) or by someone without training in HIPAA website security best practices:

Transport Encryption – Fail – Data is not encrypted during transmission

Backups – Uncertain – Most web hosting providers will backup and restore data for you. However, this assumes that the data collected is in a location backed up by the hosting company and those backups are not accessible by unauthorized personnel

Authorization – Uncertain – Depends on how the website set up

Integrity – Fail – No way to be sure that data is not tampered with or to tell if it has been

Storage Encryption – Fail – Data is never encrypted

Disposal – Uncertain – Depends on your website setup; however, some web hosts and IT departments keep data backups indefinitely and they never securely erase data

Business Associates – Fail – Many web hosting providers do not sign business associate agreements as doing so would require them to completely change their business model

What Can be Done to Guarantee Compliance?

If you have a simple corporate or informational website that has not been created from the outset with HIPAA in mind, you can be sure that adding any functions that allow ePHI to be accessed, entered into web forms, or stored is likely to result in a violation of HIPAA regulations.

Obviously, there are a large number of steps that can – and should – be taken to add the necessary security controls to ensure a website does not cause a HIPAA violation. What will work best for your organization will depend upon exactly what you are trying to accomplish with your site and in what way protected health information is presented, stored and transmitted.

Below, we discuss the seven most common problems that are encountered.

Transmission Encryption

PHI must be encrypted during transmission

The first step to secure a website is to make sure it has an SSL Certificate (i.e. the site is accessed via https://). Any page or web form that collects or displays protected health information, is used for logging in users, or uses authorization cookies, etc., must be protected by an SSL certificate and must not be accessible insecurely (i.e. there should not be an alternate insecure version of the same page that visitors can access).

The use of SSL can meet the HIPAA data transmission security requirement in terms of communications between the end user and your website; however, it is essential that the SSL configuration is robust enough and can be trusted. This requires a digital signature by a trusted Certificate Authority or CA.

Browsers include a pre-installed list of trusted CAs, known as the Trusted Root CA store. In order to be added to the Trusted Root CA store, and thus become a Certificate Authority, a company must comply with, and be audited against, security and authentication standards established by the browsers.

An SSL Certificate issued by a CA to your organization's domain/website will verify that a trusted third party has authenticated your identity. Since the browser trusts the CA, the browser will therefore trust your company website as well. The browser will also let patients and other visitors to the site know that it is secure, and your site can be browsed safely, and any data entered will be secured.

Next, what if the end user submits PHI that is collected on your website and then your website transmits that data elsewhere or stores it? These processes must also be HIPAA-compliant. We cover these in more detail below, but this will be one of your biggest challenges as it is difficult to ensure HIPAA compliance in this regard.

Backup

PHI cannot be lost – Data needs to be backed up and it must be recoverable

You must be sure that all PHI stored by your website – or collected through it – is backed up and that it can be recovered in case of an emergency or if it is accidentally deleted. Most web hosts provide this service for information stored on their servers. If your site sends information elsewhere – via email for example – then those messages must be backed up or archived and you must take care to ensure that those backups are robust, always available and accessible only by authorized people.

Note that the PHI stored in backups must also be protected in a HIPAA-compliant way — with security, authorization controls, data encryption etc.

Authorization

PHI must only be accessible by authorized personnel using unique, audited access controls

Who can access the protected health information that resides on your website or is collected through it? Your web hosting provider almost certainly can. Are they a HIPAA business associate and have you obtained an up to date business associate agreement- I.e. one that has been issued or at least revised since the introduction of the HIPAA Omnibus Rule?

If your site collects health information – such as allowing appointments to be made – and this information is sent to you or other individuals, it is important to know exactly who can access that information. This cannot be anyone with access to your email or with administrator rights to the website. Are those people trusted, have they received full training on the HIPAA Privacy and Security Rules?

If your website stores or provides access to ePHI, does it require a unique, secure login that allows only authorized personnel to access that data? Are these logins and the data accesses audited? Does the website alert the Security Officer to multiple failed login attempts? This will be up to your website designers to set up properly for you, and their work must be thoroughly tested and checked to ensure the specified controls exist and are sufficiently robust.

Integrity

PHI cannot be tampered with or altered.

Unless the information that you collect and store via your website is encrypted and/or digitally signed, there is no way to prevent it from being tampered with or to verify if tampering has occurred. It is up to your organization to determine if tamper-proofing your data is required and how to best accomplish that. Generally, using encryption for stored data can accomplish this.

Storage Encryption

PHI must be encrypted if it is stored or archived.

It is up to your organization to determine if data encryption is necessary as it is not a HIPAA requirement, instead it is an addressable issue. However, you should ask yourself: If a data breach occurred which exposed the PHI of patients, would you be able to justify to OCR inspectors your decision not to encrypt data?

If you decide to use data encryption – and it is strongly advisable to do so – you must ensure that ALL transmitted and stored protected health information is encrypted and that it can only be accessed/decrypted by individuals with the appropriate security keys. Use data encryption and your backups will be secure and all data will be properly protected (unless your security keys are stolen or divulged).

Storage encryption is especially important in any scenario where the data may be backed up or placed in locations out of your control, or in cases where a dedicated web server is not used – i.e. it is shared with other customers of the same web host. Should something unfortunate happen and a server become compromised, your liability will be significantly limited. It is, after all, not possible for PHI to be viewed without the security key, and even a hacked server will not result in a HIPAA violation if that key is not divulged.

Disposal

All PHI must be permanently erased when it is no longer required

This sounds easy. You can just delete the data when it is no longer needed. Unfortunately, deleted data can be recovered and data is frequently stored in multiple locations. It could be located in a backup, on multiple servers or in numerous files and folders.

You must consider all the places where the data could be backed up and archived. You need to ensure that all those backups are either scheduled for deletion after a finite period of time and when that occurs, they are securely and permanently erased.

Consider that any software that touches ePHI could be making backups and saving copies of your data for an indefinite period of time. It certainly helps if the data is encrypted in the backup, but if the backup is there and the keys to open that data exist, it is not really "disposed of".

It is up to you to determine how far you need to go to ensure ePHI is disposed of securely.

Business Associates

HIPAA requires you to have a signed business associate agreement with every vendor that touches ePHI.

If your website or data is located on the servers of a vendor, then HIPAA (first in HITECH and subsequently in the Omnibus Final Rule) requires you have a signed and up to date business associate agreement with them. This agreement ensures that the vendor is aware of HIPAA Privacy and Security Rules and agrees to follow them at all times.

Note that websites are complex, and no web hosting provider will be policing your website functionality and its content. They will only provide an environment that meets HIPAA requirements. It is up to you to ensure that your site is designed and managed in a way that is compliant with HIPAA.

Choosing a HIPAA-compliant provider will not make your website HIPAA compliant unless you and your designers ALSO take all of the steps to ensure that its design and functionality is complaint. This is universal unless you buy a website that is pre-designed by, and fully under the control of, a HIPAA-compliant host.

So, there are many things to do and a lot is all up to you. Of course, just because you have control over the measures you implement — or don't implement — it doesn't mean that you can make whatever choice you feel like. If you make a poor choice and a data breach occurs — or if you are audited — you are likely to be found to be willfully negligent.

Depending on the nature and extent of the breach — or severity of the HIPAA violation — this could potentially result in a fine of up to $1.5 million, per violation category, per year that the breach or violation has been allowed to persist. While your insurance policy may cover the cost of a breach, bear in mind criminal charges may also be filed in cases of willful negligence.

You therefore must carefully consider what is necessary and appropriate to suitably protect health information and the privacy of your users, and those decisions should be based on your website applications and how patient healthcare data and personal identifiers are used and transmitted.

Collecting Health Information from Website Visitors

One of the first things that doctors and medical practices like to do when they expand online is to collect patient information on their website to enable them to:

- ❖ Sign up new patients
- ❖ Schedule appointments
- ❖ Make diagnoses and recommendations about medical conditions
- ❖ Start issuing digital prescriptions

Securing the transmission of information from the patient to the website is pretty easy (it's point #1 — use website secured with a SSL Certificate). However, what do you do with the information collected via your website?

Do you store it in files on the web server to download later?

Store it in a database for download or remote access?

Email it to someone?

The third option, having the data emailed to someone, is the most popular choice because it is the easiest and requires the least additional software or infrastructure. However, it does pose a number of problems as email can be intercepted and can potentially be accessed by unauthorized individuals. So how do you make the email component meet the minimum HIPAA Privacy and Security standards and ensure that data stored or downloaded is properly protected?

Storing ePHI in files requires:

❖ The website to automatically encrypt the files

❖ Downloading the files is only possible via a secure channel (i.e. Secure FTP)

❖ The website owner receives a notification via an email that a new file is waiting

❖ Backup and secure disposal of ePHI is taken care of

Storing ePHI in a database

This allows you to write software for remote access and management of that information, however...

❖ Transmission to and from the database needs to be secure

❖ The software that provides management access must be secure and meet many HIPAA requirements governing access control and auditing

❖ Issues regarding encryption keys and database secure storage must be addressed

Option 1 is easy but requires some technical knowledge on the part of users and puts the onus of backup and disposal on them. Option 2 is better and allows more flexibility, usability and control and a centralization of all data. However, Option 2 is more technically complex and comes at a significant cost – and effort – to implement properly. There have also been many cases of databases being left exposed over the internet so care must be taken. Option 3 is easy, but how do you make the email component HIPAA compliant?

Securing Data Emailed from your Website Forms

The ideal procedure for securing your emailed data is as follows:

❖ Your secure website encrypts the submitted data (to a standard recommended by NIST) and that only a limited number of authorized individuals can open the files and view the data they contain

❖ The data is emailed to those recipients and erased from the website (or an encrypted copy is stored on the site if you prefer)

❖ The recipients receive the data and it is stored on their email server and is still encrypted

❖ The recipients can access these messages securely (over SSL) and decrypt the data either in their email program or via a web-based interface that supports decryption.

❖ The email provider takes care of backups

❖ Deleted messages will expire from backups after a finite period of time. (Obtain a signed statement from your vendor confirming this)

❖ Keep copies of all of the encrypted messages on the server instead of downloading them all, so that you are responsible for backups and make sure they are all stored in a central location.

Quickly Make Your Web Forms HIPAA-Compliant

There are a number of HIPAA-compliant providers who can help you achieve this. For example, JotForm offers a HIPAA compliant web form platform to allow you to collect data from your website in a way that is both automatically HIPAA-compliant and does not require any programming on your part. JotForm allows you to collect data on a website and has the following features:

❖ Encrypts data as it is entered into the form and data is transferred and stored using end-to-end encryption

❖ Storage of encrypted data on HIPAA compliant servers protected by multiple layers of security

❖ HIPAA-compliant access controls

❖ Alerts are generated when forms are completed, but form data is not sent in email notifications

❖ The solution integrates with HIPAA compliant services such as Dropbox, Google Sheets, and Google Drive for downloading form data

❖ Obtain digital signatures from patients to confirm identity

Internal IT Network Security

Network security is a vital element of HIPAA compliance. You must ensure your facility has robust multi-layered information security protections that safeguards ePHI and keeps it secure at all times. Measures must be introduced that protect against intrusion, offer extended connectivity, allow easy incorporation of software packages and bespoke programs and permit secure backups of data while eliminating downtime.

There are a number of companies that offer HIPAA-compliant networks for healthcare providers, health plans, clearinghouses and other covered entities, such as the Medical-grade networks offered by Cisco and SonicWALL healthcare information solutions from Dell. These scalable solutions provide the framework that allows HIPAA-compliant interactions between healthcare professionals, processes, applications and software and hardware components.

While these network solutions can be invaluable for healthcare providers looking to comply with HIPAA regulations and the Meaningful Use Incentive program, they are not a universal solution that will guarantee compliance with the HIPAA Privacy and Security Rules. There are many potential areas for HIPAA violations to occur, especially with the following devices and security solutions, which pose a particularly high risk of ePHI exposure. As such, they are the most likely source of intrusion and are all potential areas that hackers can use to gain access to healthcare databases:

- ❖ Routers
- ❖ Firewalls
- ❖ Virtual Private Networks (VPNs)
- ❖ Wireless Access
- ❖ Windows-Based Email and Web Servers

Each of the above must be thoroughly checked by conducting a comprehensive risk analysis, and each item must be certified as being secure and compliant with HIPAA regulations. HIPAA requires organizations to implement a multi-layered security system and the first layer is usually the router, not the firewall. A router helps to protect a firewall from attack, not the other way round.

Routers

While a firewall will protect a network against intrusion, a router can offer some protection for the firewall and ease the burden placed on it to stop unauthorized access to internal healthcare systems. Routers are not specifically mentioned in HIPAA, but that does not mean they are not a major risk.

A router filters unwanted external traffic and acts as a packet filter which stops the firewall from having to analyze each packet presented to the router; however, routers must be configured for the healthcare environment where they are used.

Each router is supplied with a set of security controls by the manufacturer, and in a home environment, this may be sufficient, but in a healthcare environment, where targeted attacks are likely, they do not offer the required level of protection.

An Access Control List (ACL) should be used. This allows security filtering and blocks to be placed on IP addresses, while extended ACLs also deny or permit packets based on packet header information, protocols or port numbers.

The golden rule for securing routers is to configure them to deny all packets unless they are specifically designated to be allowed, rather than to allow all packets unless they are specifically denied. It is also a good best practice to close any ports which are not in use and you must change default login credentials and set strong passwords.

Routers must also be thoroughly tested. Penetration testing software such as Nmap, Netcat, Nessus and Enum can be used to achieve this and determine whether the router has been configured correctly. It is also essential that routers are monitored for intrusion attempts and they must be configured to automatically generate audit logs – which must be checked frequently for signs that access has been attempted or allowed.

It is all too easy to concentrate on the technical aspect of network security, but the routers themselves must be protected from tampering. It is a quick and easy process to reset routers to factory standards and undo protections, so they must also be physically secured and access to the location where they are housed must be controlled.

Firewalls

The second line of defense against unauthorized access to healthcare computer systems is the firewall. A firewall offers packet-level security and acts like a router in this regard, denying or allowing access. A firewall must be placed between the internal servers and the external environment, such as between an internal server and the connection to the internet, and also between web and mail servers and the internet.

There are numerous types of firewall that can be used as detailed below, with each offering benefits and disadvantages.

Stateful Application Gateway Proxy – Opens up packets, inspects them and rewrites them. These are secure, but slow.

Appliance Firewall – Appliance firewalls are easier to install, although they are more expensive.

Packet Filters – While effective and offering a high degree of protection, they can be complicated to set up and next to useless if not configured correctly.

Application Proxies – These are secure, offer a high degree of protection and are flexible, although they use considerable system resources and have a tendency to be slow.

Stateful Inspection Firewalls – Correct configuration is essential, but these firewalls are faster and offer a compromise between a secure application proxy and the less secure packet filtering.

Software Firewalls – Offer an increased level of protection, although they are insufficient protection on their own and should never be used without a network firewall.

As with routers, firewalls should block all access to the external environment and prevent access to internal systems unless they are specifically allowed and their configurations must be tested, there must be automatic reporting of failed and granted access and procedures should be developed to ensure that the firewall is always active.

Virtual Private Networks (VPNs)

A Virtual Private Network or VPN can be used to allow users to access internal systems through a secure tunnel via public networks, such as accessing internal systems via the internet. They also incorporate a system of authenticating users and encrypt data transferred through them.

Different levels of security exist, and while not perfect, the IPSec protocol offers an appropriate degree of protection provided that the VPN has been correctly configured at both ends: The user end and the internal servers which are accessed via the VPN.

A VPN offers some protection, but alone this is insufficient and other security measures must also be used. One important point is that users must not be connected to the internal network via the VPN at the same time as being connected to the internet unless a personal firewall is installed on the device and is active. Audit logs should also be automatically generated to ensure intrusion attempts can be identified. VPN software must also be kept up to date and only the latest version of the software should be used.

Wireless Access

Wireless networks allow medical professionals to connect to internal networks via hand-held and other portable devices, allowing them instant access to ePHI such as medical records and test results. Since no cables are needed, a wireless network allows data to be accessed from any area of the facility, such as treatment or examination rooms.

However, wireless network access is inherently insecure. The signals are sent out in all directions, including outside of the facility itself, and offer a way into the internal network. Because of the high risk, healthcare organizations should opt for a closed network and should take the following actions:

The wireless router should be positioned in a location that restricts the distance outside the facility the signal can be sent. I.e., not placing it next to an external wall or window, instead locating it centrally in the building

Wireless networks should be configured using WEP (Wireless Encryption Protocol). This should not be confused with other more robust data encryption methods used to protect the data itself, as WEP is not completely secure and must be used with other LAN security mechanisms

- ❖ Change factory default logins and passwords. Use long alphanumeric passwords to offer a greater level of security

- ❖ Use access lists which control who can connect to the network

- ❖ Change the SSID along with the default login details

- ❖ Disable DHCP and only use assigned IP addresses on WAPs and on the devices used to connect to them

- ❖ Only allow access to wireless networks via a VPN

Windows-Based Web Servers

Windows based web servers are easy to hack, especially if patches and updates are not installed. Security holes do exist, although Microsoft plugs these holes quickly once they are identified. Microsoft does this by issuing updates and patches. Servers should be configured to update and install these automatically if possible. If not, it is essential for IT teams to keep on top of patching.

If a server is not patched it will be particularly vulnerable to attack and may not only result in the data on the server being exposed, but a hacked server can be used to connect to other servers in the facility.

A good best practice is to make sure all default configurations are changed, including scripts, the location of the web folder and default system permissions. All default users must be removed from the server as these are one of the main methods used to improperly access servers.

Procedures must be developed governing the creation of passwords. Only strong passwords should be permitted, while users should be required to change these periodically, say, every 6 months. Rate limiting should also be set up to reduce the potential for brute force attacks.

Posix and OS/2 should be removed and NetBIOS disabled. O/S, HTML and FTP folders should also be separated, using hard drive partitions or even better, separate hard drives for each.

You must also ensure that antivirus software is installed, that it is automatically updated with new definitions and routine scans of the server should be conducted to check for viruses and malware which may have bypassed other security controls.

Email Security

What are the HIPAA Rules for Email Encryption?

The HIPAA email encryption rules do not exclusively apply to emails, but to all communications which contain protected health information in electronic form. Therefore, attachments to emails, SMS and IMs are governed by the HIPAA rules for email encryption, but not faxes or voicemail messages (unless they are saved in electronic form after they have been received, in which case the Security Rule provision for protected health information at rest applies).

What HIPAA actually says about email encryption is that covered entities must "implement a mechanism to encrypt and decrypt electronic Protected Health Information", and most communication experts agree that healthcare organizations who want to facilitate the communication of protected health information by email should double their encryption protection, so that encrypted communications are sent over an encrypted connection "just to be on the safe side".

Why the Communication of Protected Health Information by Email is Insecure

The experts´ wariness about HIPAA email encryption rules is based on several possible scenarios in which a breach of protected health information could occur when the data is communicated by email.

For example:

When emails are sent using public FTP (File Transfer Protocol), copies of the emails will remain on routing servers indefinitely with no possibility of an organization being able to delete them if a breach of protected health information is identified

There is no possibility of retracting an email containing ePHI if it has been sent to the wrong person, or to remotely delete emails if an authorized user loses a mobile device from which ePHI has been communicated

There is also the logistical issue that each authorized user would have to install encryption/decryption software on all the mobile devices and desktop computers they would use for the communication of ePHI by email, and that the software would have to operate across all platforms

Furthermore, any solution that is implemented to comply with the HIPAA rules for email encryption would also have to have administrative controls to monitor access to ePHI. You must also ensure that the policies developed to comply with the HIPAA email encryption rules are being adhered to

An Alternative to Encrypted Emails

There is an alternative to encrypted emails, and that is to use a secure messaging platform. This works by allowing access to protected health information through a software-as-a-service "On Demand" app. The app can conveniently be used from any desktop computer or mobile device, while administrative controls safeguard the integrity of ePHI.

Access to ePHI is only available to authorized users who are assigned a unique username and PIN, and whose activity on the secure messaging platform is monitored with access reports and audit logs automatically generated.

As all activity is contained within a private network, should a breach of ePHI be identified, administrators can remotely delete a message – unlike when the communication of ePHI occurs via email – or remotely wipe the user from the system if their personal mobile device is lost or stolen.

Secure messaging apps have been purposefully designed with the end-user in mind; and medical professionals, business associates and third-party service providers should find the text-like interface familiar and easy to use, making it less likely that they would revert to alternative insecure channels to communicate ePHI.

The Benefits of Secure Messaging Over Secure Emails

Research conducted on mobile device users has shown that messaging is by far the most popular form of mobile communication, with 92% of mobile users preferring it over email because of the speed of delivery. A further fact, revealed in a 2012 survey, was that respondents considered text communications to be more urgent than emails – and required an immediate response, rather than delaying an answer until it was more convenient.

In a healthcare environment, the speed of response can have substantial benefits to patients, plus there are additional benefits for medical professionals and healthcare organizations when secure messaging is used, such as accelerating patient concerns, making faster diagnoses, delivering lab results more quickly and efficiently and assisting in the administration of medical treatment.

Secure messaging apps have a message forwarding feature which enables multiple parties to collaborate securely about the care provided to a patient

Authorized users receive delivery notifications and read receipts that confirm their messages have been received and which eliminate phone tag

Secure messages can be assigned a lifespan and delete automatically after a pre-determined period of time

A "search by name" facility helps eliminate the risk of messaging errors often seen with encrypted email, and accelerates secure communications between medical professionals

Each of these features helps to streamline workflows, increase productivity and improve the standard of patient healthcare in a cost-effective manner, while maintaining the integrity of protected health information at all times.

Text Messages and Replacing Pagers

Finding a pager replacement for hospitals has become a priority since legislation was enacted in the Health Insurance Portability and Accountability Act (HIPAA) to increase patients´ privacy and the security of ePHI.

Pagers are inherently insecure channels of communication for transmitting ePHI, as there is no accountability for messages that are sent by pager and no automated auditing option. Pager messages can be missed, sent to the wrong recipient or intercepted by a third party.

Other issues of concern – and why finding a replacement for hospital pagers has become a priority – are the limitations of paging systems. It is not possible to share images via a pager, thus making them impractical for healthcare organizations that want to create a team-based care environment and, due to the restricted coverage of paging systems, they are inappropriate for medical professionals working off site.

What HIPAA has to Say about Communicating ePHI via a Pager

The HIPAA Security Rule introduced administrative, physical and technical safeguards that stipulate how ePHI should be stored and communicated. In order to be compliant with the HIPAA Security Rule, healthcare organizations must be able to identify the sources of all ePHI that is created and monitor how it is maintained, accessed and communicated.

As healthcare organizations have no control over what is communicated via a pager, it is not possible to comply with HIPAA when a paging system is implemented in a hospital environment. So, although HIPAA does not specifically mention anything about communicating ePHI via a pager, healthcare organizations using paging systems have two options if they are to become HIPAA-compliant – either prohibit the communication of ePHI through the paging system or find a pager replacement for hospitals.

Using Existing Technology as a Pager Replacement

The most obvious solution is to use existing technology as a pager replacement. Numerous surveys have shown that up to 80% of healthcare professionals use a smartphone or other personal mobile device in hospitals and harnessing this existing channel of communication is a cost-effective way of dealing with the pager issue, provided of course that any messaging conducted between personal mobile devices is HIPAA-compliant.

HIPAA compliance can be assured by using secure texting platforms. Secure texting replicates the speed and convenience of SMS messaging, but has the controls in place to prevent potential breaches of ePHI. Secure texting also has the benefits of limitless coverage and the ability to exchange images and foster a collaborative healthcare environment. It can also be used by healthcare organizations to qualify for Meaningful Use incentive payments.

Secure Texting as a Replacement for Hospital Pagers

Secure texting requires everybody connected to the healthcare organization´s network to download a secure texting app. The app has a text-like interface which will be familiar to any healthcare professional that has a mobile phone, and it enables them to communicate ePHI securely, share information with colleagues and receive notifications that their communications have been received and read – thus overcoming issues such as accountability and recipient delivery and eliminating productivity-reducing phone tag.

The platform through which all secure texts pass has administrative controls that have the ability to remotely retract and delete text messages, assign message lifespans – so that messages are deleted and archived automatically – time out a mobile device if it has been inactive for a period of time, and remove a user from the organization´s network if the mobile device is lost or stolen or their employment is terminated.

In addition to ensuring compliant usage of the secure messaging solution, the administrative controls also produce audit reports to comply with the HIPAA safeguards for monitoring how ePHI is maintained, accessed and communicated.

TigerText is a leading provider of secure texting solutions, and their platform has allowed many healthcare providers to replace their pager systems entirely. To date, the secure messaging system has been implemented in more than 4,000 medical facilities. As a HIPAA-compliant pager replacement, a secure texting solution can lead to streamlined workflows, increased productivity and enhanced standards of patient care while securing communications and data transmissions.

Advantages of a modern secure messaging solution as a replacement for pagers can include integration of secure messages with the hospital´s answering service and EHRs while staff communications are streamlined, potentially saving thousands of dollars, an accountable message delivery and receipt system, enhanced clinical workflows, accelerated patient hand-offs, and implementation of a priority messaging channel in order that offsite staff members could escalate patient concerns securely and deliver patient care more quickly. With the ability to attach files and images to secure messages, workflows can be accelerated and offsite staff members able to spend more time providing medical care to patients.

9. The Costs and Benefits of HIPAA Compliance

The Impact of HIPAA

The Health Insurance Portability and Accountability Act was a landmark bill that introduced sweeping changes in the healthcare industry. The bill was originally introduced with two main aims: To allow individuals to maintain their health insurance between jobs and ensure the security and confidentiality of patient information and healthcare data. New standards were also introduced covering the electronic transmission and storage of data relating to patient health information.

The bill limits the pre-existing condition restrictions that a group health insurance arrangement can enforce, meaning that as long as individuals have continuous coverage, a group policy cannot exclude a pre-existing condition.

HIPAA has made a considerable difference to how healthcare data is stored, transmitted and safeguarded. As the healthcare industry has moved from physical records to electronic versions, the risk of that data being exposed or viewed by unauthorized individuals has increased considerably. HIPAA is therefore an essential piece of legislation that forces healthcare providers and other covered entities to implement a wide range of safeguards to protect the privacy of patients and health plan members.

For patients and health plan members the benefits of HIPAA-compliance are clear. Data is protected and insurance coverage secured. A HIPAA-compliant healthcare organization also inspires confidence and trust and assures the public that the organization in question is committed to protecting the privacy of its patients and plan members.

However, for organizations covered by HIPAA the benefits may not be immediately apparent, and it is all too easy to focus on the disadvantages that come from HIPAA. Becoming compliant involves committing a considerable amount of resources to improving security and protecting privacy, it requires greater investment in software and hardware, and it carries a considerable administrative burden and the cost of HIPAA-compliance can be considerable.

Those costs must be found from somewhere and some medical professional argue that that money diverted to compliance would be better spent on improving the healthcare services provided to patients. However, even with the cost, the advantages of HIPAA far outweigh the disadvantages.

The Benefits of Compliance

The main benefit of healthcare providers, health plans and healthcare clearinghouses becoming

HIPAA-compliant is that it is the only way that these organizations will be able to avoid multi-million-dollar fines. Becoming HIPAA-compliant is, after all, not a choice but a requirement.

While enforcement was been lax in the early years of the legislation, since 2009 the Office for Civil Rights, along with state Attorneys General, have been policing HIPAA more rigorously and major fines are being issued to organizations that have suffered data breaches as a result of a failure to implement the appropriate safeguards to protect data. Fines can also be issued for noncompliance, even in the absence of a data breach.

There is a considerable cost advantage to becoming HIPAA-compliant. While it may involve a significant initial cost — and ongoing costs to stay HIPAA-compliant — they pale into insignificance compared to the costs associated with data breaches and regulatory fines.

It is not only fines from the Office for Civil Rights and state Attorneys General that covered entities have to cover. The cost of issuing breach notifications and damage mitigation can run into millions of dollars as well as the legal costs from dealing with lawsuits.

The mega data breach that affected Anthem Inc., in February 2015 exposed 78.8 million records. The initial estimates of the cost of the breach were well in excess of 100 million. The reality however is likely to be far worse. Some industry experts have predicted that the final cost of the data breach – which will not be known for some time – could well rise to $1 billion. These estimates do not even take into consideration the loss of revenue that may come as a result of consumers losing trust in the insurer's ability to safeguard their healthcare data.

There are many more benefits to healthcare organizations than cost savings, many of which come from the transition from physical records to EHRs.

Compliance with the Health Insurance Portability and Accountability Act:

- ❖ Helps covered entities prevent data breaches and restricts the damage caused when they do occur
- ❖ Ensures that in the event of an emergency, healthcare services can still be provided
- ❖ Makes sure healthcare data cannot be lost or accidentally deleted
- ❖ Improves efficiency
- ❖ Improves access to healthcare information
- ❖ Streamlines the provision of medical services
- ❖ Allows organizations to qualify for Meaningful Use financial incentives
- ❖ Improves patient confidence and trust

When HIPAA was introduced, one of the aims was to create a simpler, more standardized healthcare system that would eventually lower health care costs while reducing errors through safe, universally accepted electronic communication of healthcare transactions.

It has now been more than 20 years since the introduction of the legislation and while the jury

may still be out on the effectiveness of the bill –
and whether HIPAA has been worth the time,
energy, and financial investment – consumers have
certainly received many important benefits and,
over time, so will the organizations that implement
the standards necessary to comply with HIPAA.

10. HIPAA Training

While training employees on HIPAA requirements is absolutely necessary, the requirements laid out by the legislation regarding training are vague. This is in part due to the fact HIPAA covers a broad range of covered entities and their business associates. The training requirements for a healthcare clearinghouse will naturally be different to those of a healthcare provider, so it is left to the discretion of each covered entity to determine what is reasonable and appropriate.

Training, in some form, is required under the administrative requirements of the HIPAA Privacy Rule and is a requirement of the administrative safeguard of the HIPAA Security Rule. Neither provide very comprehensive information on what is required in terms of training. They state that training should be provided "as necessary and appropriate for members of the workforce to carry out their functions" (HIPAA Privacy Rule) and that covered entities and business associates should "implement a security awareness and training program for all members of the workforce" (HIPAA Security Rule).

Regrettably, this lack of certainty regarding HIPAA training does lend itself to confusion. Despite the lack of clear rules, should a breach of Protected Health Information (PHI) occur and it is found that staff weren't adequately trained, the covered entity and business associates may be issued with a fine by the Office for Civil Rights (OCR).

Objectives of HIPAA Training

To prevent such a breach happening, it is essential that regular risk analyses are conducted by covered entities and business associates. These will help to establish the role each employee with respect to PHI. This can help ensure that each employee gets training appropriate to his/her role.

Covered entities should tailor security awareness and training programs for the role of each employee, manager, associate etc., that come in contact with PHI. For complex roles, many training sessions may be required.

Providing training can be costly and time-consuming, which is often off-putting. It is, however, necessary. We recommend that training sessions are offered in shorter, frequent sessions rather than one long session. This way, employees are more likely to stay focused and retain critical information.

Training Tips

To help covered entities and their business associates navigate the confusing world of HIPAA compliance training, we have compiled a simple list of best practices for employee training.

Do try to keep training sessions short. This will make employees more likely to retain information and thus help prevent further breaches. Remember: Ignorance is not considered an excuse for PHI breaches or HIPAA violations.

Do provide regular training sessions. Each can focus on a different aspect of training, update staff on new developments, or even just remind employees of the most important aspects of HIPAA Rules.

Do inform employees of the dangers of a PHI breach. These can include fines and legal action for the covered entity, privacy violations for patients, and even criminal charges in some situations. Such information can help highlight the need for HIPAA compliance.

Do include all levels of management in training. Everybody needs a refresher from time to time, and a lack of training provided to higher levels reflects poorly on the covered entity in an audit.

Don't forget to make clear records of when the training occurred, who was involved and what information was handed out. If OCR carries out an investigation or an audit, this information will need to be provided.

Don't just read passages from HIPAA. Explain legal jargon and summarize important pieces of information. Try to ensure that participants both know the required legislation but also understand how to enact it in their day-to-day roles.

Don't go into the history of HIPAA – it is not essential information and is likely to cause participants to lose focus before you even begin. Having so much information thrown at you before you even get into the important information will alienate employees.

Sample Curriculum

Designing a training course can be complicated, and it can be difficult to decide what is appropriate for different employees. Here we describe a sample HIPAA training curriculum, which can be tailored as needed. Some modules – such as the Introduction to HIPAA – are core elements for all employees, whilst others are more suitable for those in specific roles. Who receives what training is at the discretion of the covered entity.

1. Introduction to HIPAA – This should include a brief overview of HIPAA legislation, as well as detail the main aspects of the act. This should not, however, include a long introduction to the history of HIPAA.

   a. *Why is HIPAA needed?* – Though this may seem intuitive, there is no harm in reminding employees of why acts such as HIPAA are required. This can include case-studies of recent incidents where HIPAA was breached.

   b. *HIPAA terminology* – HIPAA is a complex piece of legal documentation. It would be unreasonable to expect all employees to understand the terminology, so providing a "glossary" of common terms (e.g. "covered entity") will be hugely beneficial.

c. *Applicability of HIPAA* – Knowing who has to abide by HIPAA policy is essential in ensuring compliance.

2. Covered Entities – A covered entity is an entity that creates healthcare information or uses healthcare data for providing healthcare, payment for healthcare, or performs healthcare operations and conducts healthcare transactions electronically. They must be HIPAA compliant, meaning they must ensure the confidentiality, integrity, and availability of PHI.

   a. *Examples of covered entities* – Generally, any hospital, medical practitioner, healthcare clearinghouse or billing company are considered to be covered entities.

   b. *Are employers covered entities?* – Generally, employers are not considered to be covered entities, though they often have healthcare records of their employees.

3. Business Associates – Business Associates are any organization or individual that is contracted by the covered entity to perform a service that requires contact with PHI. They must also be HIPAA-compliant, and thus any business associates must train their employees on HIPAA requirements.

   a. *Types of business associates* – "business associate" essentially includes any external body hired by the covered entity to perform a service.

This can range from management consultants to accountants and software providers. As long as they have access to PHI, they must be HIPAA-compliant.

b. *Business Associate Agreement* – Before providing access to PHI to a business associate, a covered entity must ensure that the business associate signs a Business Associate Agreement. This is a legal document confirming they understand their responsibilities with respect to PHI and HIPAA.

4. What is PHI? – Under the HIPAA Privacy Rule, certain classes of information are deemed to be "protected" and must remain confidential. They cannot be transmitted to or accessed by unauthorized personnel. Any employee that comes into contact with such information must be trained to identify it and treat it accordingly.

   a. *Examples of PHI* – PHI includes one of 18 identifiers in combination with health information in the past, present, and future that is used for providing healthcare, payment for healthcare, or healthcare operations.

5. HIPAA Rules – Since it was originally written, many aspects of HIPAA have been amended. This includes the addition of many "rules" that address specific aspects of patient and data privacy. Most employees will deal with specific rules or aspects of the rules, so the next section can be tailored to their need.

a. *Privacy Rule* – The Privacy Rule defined PHI and also instructed covered entities on allowable uses and disclosures. It also gave patients privacy rights, including the right not to disclose private health care information to health insurers. The Privacy Rule also includes the Minimum Necessary Rule, which stipulates that only the minimum amount of information required to complete a task may be passed on to another authorized entity.

b. *Security Rule* – The Security Rule addresses electronic PHI (ePHI). It outlines the administrative, physical and technical safeguards needed to protect health data.

c. *Enforcement Rule* – To help ensure that HIPAA is being followed, the Enforcement Rule was introduced. It outlines the penalties for non-compliance, and gives the Department of Health and Human Services the ability to prosecute for HIPAA violations.

d. *Breach Notification Rule* – The Breach Notification Rule stipulates that a covered entity or business associate has 30 days after the discovery of a breach to notify the OCR, patients and the media.

e. *Omnibus Final Rule* – The most recent addition to HIPAA, the Omnibus Rule addresses a wide range of areas and implemented the requirements of the HITECH Act.

6. HIPAA Password Policies

   a. *Password strength* – Passwords should contain a good mixture of upper- and lower-case letters, as well as numbers and special characters where permitted. Longer passwords are better. Check NIST advice and set policies and train employees accordingly.

7. HITECH Act – The Health Information Technology for Economic and Clinical Health Act was introduced to help the healthcare sector adapt to the modern age.

   a. *Meaningful use* – Under HITECH, those holding electronic health records (EHR) must show that there is legitimate purpose for holding onto healthcare records. Initially optional, it is now mandatory for all healthcare providers.

   b. *HITECH and HIPAA* – Though separate from HIPAA, it is closely related to the act and acts to reinforcement. HIPAA Rules. Whilst HIPAA focuses on all aspects of privacy, the HITECH Act has special focus on digital health records.

8. Exceptions to HIPAA Privacy – Children and Minors

   a. *Cases of abuse* – Unfortunately, working in the healthcare profession, medics may come across distressing cases. If a covered entity has reasonable grounds to believe that a minor is being abused/neglected, the covered entity can choose not to disclose the patient's health information with the legal guardian. They may also inform the police or child services.

b. *Independent minors* – If a minor has emancipated him/herself from their legal guardian, they must be treated as a legal adult.

c. *Legal requirements* – If a court decides that someone other than the minor's legal parent or guardian must make their medical decisions, a third party may access the child's healthcare data.

9. Threats to Privacy

a. *Cybercrime* – Regrettably, healthcare data is an increasingly prominent target for cybercriminals as it has huge value on the black market. Thus, cybercrime – primarily in the form of hacking – poses a huge threat to the data privacy. Adopting some of the aforementioned policies and practices can help lessen the threat.

b. *Human error* – All employees will make mistakes from time to time – it is completely normal. However, when this threatens patient privacy, such mistakes can have resounding consequences. It is essential that employees understand the potential dangers of HIPAA non-compliance and that they understand that they must report breaches.

10.   Penalties for Non-Compliance – For any piece of legislation to have authority, there must be adequate penalties to act as a deterrent. HIPAA is no exception. Ensuring employees have adequate understanding of the potential penalties for HIPAA non-compliance can help prevent breaches.

   a. *Administrative fines* – Financial penalties for HIPAA non-compliance be as high as $1.5 million per violation category per year. Penalty amounts depend on the level of culpability.

   b. *Personal fines* – If an individual violated HIPAA and there was malicious intent behind their actions, they can face a personal fine of up to $250,000.

   c. *Jail sentences* – In some instances, if a violation is deemed sufficiently severe, an individual may receive a jail sentence of up to 10 years.

11.   Security Awareness – All employees must be given security awareness training to help them identity threats and vulnerabilities to the confidentiality, integrity, and availability of PHI.

   a. *Phishing awareness* – It is important to train employees how to recognize phishing emails and the actions they should and should not take when such an email is received

HIPAA Compliance Training: Summary

The phrasing of HIPAA legislation means it is up to covered entities and their business associates to determine how best to provide training to employees. Ultimately, so long as sufficient training is provided to allow employees understand how to prevent PHI breaches, privacy violations, and be aware of patient rights it should be adequate. Training should also be tailored to the role of individual employees, which both maximizes efficiency and increases the likelihood of knowledge retention. The sample curriculum supplied here is a good base from which a full training course can be developed.

11. HIPAA Resources

Office for Civil Rights
http://www.hhs.gov/ocr/office/index.html

OCR Breach Reporting
https://ocrportal.hhs.gov/ocr/breach/wizard_breach.jsf

HIPAA Security Rule
http://www.hhs.gov/ocr/privacy/hipaa/administrative/securit
yrule/index.html

HIPAA Security Rule Guidance
http://www.hhs.gov/ocr/privacy/hipaa/administrative/securit
yrule/securityruleguidance.html

Security Risk Assessments
http://www.healthit.gov/providers-professionals/security-
risk-assessment

HHS – Final Guidance – Risk Assessments
http://www.hhs.gov/ocr/privacy/hipaa/administrative/securit
yrule/rafinalguidancepdf.pdf

Security Standards – Final Rule
http://www.hhs.gov/ocr/privacy/hipaa/administrative/securit
yrule/securityrulepdf.pdf

Security and Electronic Signature Standards
http://www.hhs.gov/ocr/privacy/hipaa/administrative/securit
yrule/srnprm.pdf

HIPAA Privacy Rule
http://www.hhs.gov/ocr/privacy/hipaa/administrative/privacy
rule/index.html

Notice of Privacy Practices
http://www.hhs.gov/ocr/privacy/hipaa/modelnotices.html

Health Information Privacy Rights
http://www.hhs.gov/ocr/privacy/index.html

De-identification of PHI
http://www.hhs.gov/ocr/privacy/hipaa/understanding/covere
dentities/De-identification/deidentificationworkshop2010.html

HIPAA Breach Notification Rule
http://www.hhs.gov/ocr/privacy/hipaa/administrative/breach
notificationrule/index.html

Example Breach Notification Letter
http://www.hhs.gov/ocr/privacy/hipaa/enforcement/audit/sa
mple-ocr_notification_ltr.pdf

HIPAA Enforcement
http://www.hhs.gov/ocr/privacy/hipaa/enforcement/index.ht
ml

HIPAA Resolution Agreements
http://www.hhs.gov/ocr/privacy/hipaa/enforcement/example
s/index.html

HIPAA Enforcement – State Attorneys General
http://www.hhs.gov/ocr/privacy/hipaa/enforcement/sag/inde
x.html

HIPAA Omnibus Rule
http://www.hhs.gov/news/press/2013pres/01/20130117b.ht
ml

HIPAA and the HITECH Act
http://www.gpo.gov/fdsys/pkg/FR-2013-01-25/pdf/2013-
01073.pdf

Business Associate Agreements
http://www.hhs.gov/ocr/privacy/hipaa/understanding/covere
dentities/contractprov.html

Business Associate Guidance
http://www.hhs.gov/ocr/privacy/hipaa/faq/business_associat
es/

HIPAA Compliance Audits

http://www.hhs.gov/ocr/privacy/hipaa/enforcement/audit/ind
ex.html

HIPAA, FERPA and Student Health Records

http://www.hhs.gov/ocr/privacy/hipaa/understanding/covere
dentities/hipaaferpajointguide.pdf

HIPAA and Digital Copiers

https://www.ftc.gov/tips-advice/business-
center/guidance/copier-data-security-guide-businesses

HIPAA in Emergency Situations

http://www.hhs.gov/ocr/privacy/hipaa/understanding/special/
emergency/emergencysituations.pdf

HIPAA and Workplace Wellness Programs

http://www.hhs.gov/ocr/privacy/hipaa/understanding/covere
dentities/wellness/index.html

Also Available from the Publisher

The Basics of HIPAA Compliance: A Guide for Employees

A brief but comprehensive overview of HIPAA regulations, intended as a quick-reference for all staff and employees and suitable for use as an introductory training course for existing staff and new hires.

The HIPAA Compliance Toolkit

Professionally prepared compliance program addresses all major regulatory requirements imposed by HIPAA and its regulations.

Each module contains detailed instructions, extensive documentation, and templates for all necessary compliance documents.

Security Risk Assessment Module
BA/Vendor/Subcontractor Module
Education and Training Module
Privacy and Security Policy Module

www.apexlegalpublishing.com

Made in the USA
Monee, IL
18 February 2023

28094202R00085